THE FASTING PLAN

USE INTERMITTENT FASTING TO GET LEAN AND STAY LEAN FOREVER

NICK HOLT

Why I Wrote This Book

If you're reading this right now, you are just like me. I don't care where you're from, what you look like and what is going on in your life. You're like me because deep down, we both want to improve our lives. It's engrained in our nature as human beings.

I've spent 23 years of my life in the fitness world. I've tried just about every single diet you can imagine, and I've competed in over 40 different fitness competitions. I've been fat. I've been lean. I've been happy about the way I look, and I've been depressed about it. We all want to feel good about ourselves and we all want to live long, healthy lives.

There are tons of dieting books out there. Yet, there are so many people that are still out of shape and who can't seem to find a solution that is easy to stick with for long-term results. Over the last three years, I've used fasting to get in the best shape I've been in my entire life. The habits I've been able to develop make dieting almost effortless. Friends of mine started asking me about my diet and one after another started using my fasting techniques and have seen incredible results. Soon after, Kris Gethin, one of my best friends, lit a fire under my ass by telling me I needed to put everything I've been doing into a complete program. Hence, The Fasting Plan was born.

The greatest feeling I can get in life is knowing I've been able to help someone in some way, shape or form. I've had friends try this program and tell me how much better they look and feel. They are able to get in shape and maintain it with ease. Watching them strut around with this new confidence has made a huge impact on my life. It has taken a lot of guts for me to get out of my comfort zone and write this book, but I've done it anyway because of the deep satisfaction I've already received. Even if only one person changes their life with this program, I would be eternally grateful for getting the opportunity to help someone.

WHY YOU SHOULD READ THIS BOOK

Imagine a diet that allows you to eat as much as you want while helping you get lean and stay lean all year long. No sacrificing social life, career commitments or obligations. No carrying around a cooler to and from work, eating pre-made meals out of Tupperware. Just a few simple guidelines to follow and—boom! More energy! More happiness! More freedom and confidence!

I've created such a program and it's called The Fasting Plan. It will show you everything you need to know about fasting and how to use it to get in the best physical shape and stay that way... FOREVER.

This program will give you all the tools, tips, tactics and tricks you need to turn your body into a fat-burning machine.

You'll learn:

- How to fast

- How to break your fast

- The difference between all the different forms of fasting and what works best

- The most common fasting myths

- What types of food to eat and when

- Why fasting is great for fat-loss and what the studies are saying

- The best recipes for breaking your fast

- How to deal with hunger and conquer your cravings

- The most common questions answered

- And much more!

This program is action-packed with value and I'm very excited to share it with you. Thank you for taking the time to check out The Fasting Plan.

Sincerely yours,

Nick

IMPORANT NOTE

Read this before you begin!

For your convenience, I've tailored this program specifically for two different types of people. Read the following questions below. The way you use TFP will depend on what your answers are!

QUESTION 1:

Are you the type of person who wants to learn WHY this plan works so well and WHAT you need to know about it before executing it?

QUESTION: 2:

Are you the type of person who just wants to skip ahead and get started already? Do you want a step-by-step series of tips and strategies you can follow right away to show you HOW you can take action right now?

If you are the type of person that is more in line with question one, I have you covered. Go ahead and start reading this book from the beginning to the end. I'll cover why the fasting plan is important and explain in detailed fashion everything you need to know about fasting and show you how to use it to burn fat and get in shape as quickly as possible.

If you are the type of person that is more in line with question two, I have your back too! In this case, I've developed a quick start guide for you. In this quick start guide, you'll be shown exactly what to do to start fasting today. This will expedite things for you and allow you to jump right in to The Fasting Plan!

*Just remember, I highly recommend you go back and read the entire book because it will give you a much better understanding of fasting and how it works with your body. Doing this is what I believe will ensure success for LIFE!

The quick start guide can be found in the resources section in the back of the book.

Table of Contents

Part 1: What You Need To Know About Intermittent Fasting

Why are you reading this right now? What is the reason you picked up this book? You have to answer that question for yourself. There's a very high chance that you're here right now at this very moment because you know there is something about your life that has to change. Something is missing. Something is deficient. The way you are living your life is no longer suitable for your course of action. You've failed too many times and hit roadblocks over and over again and don't know where to go or what to do. You've looked in the mirror too many times and haven't smiled. You want to change your current situation and move from where you are to some place better. You want to move up and improve your life by growing, helping, giving and conquering your deepest convictions. Before you begin this journey with me, you need to fuel yourself with the right reasons to move forward. So, do me a favor. Follow this action step right now: Take out a piece of paper or use a note in your phone and answer these questions.

1.   Why do I want to improve my health?

2.   If I did improve my health, what value would it add to my life?

3.   Who would it impact and how would it make their lives better?

Answering these three questions will give you a solid reason why you need to do this. It will be your reason for grinding this shit out when it gets tough. Because, I'm here to tell you: This program kicks ass, but it won't be easy. Nothing worth having ever is. Have I scared you off yet? If so, good. I don't want people to do this program or read this book if they aren't willing to sacrifice who they are for who they will become. To make a positive change in your life, you need to be willing to put in the work.

Here's another thought for you:

No matter what you want to accomplish in life, you can't do it unless you are healthy. Stop and think about this. Now imagine what you can accomplish if you are healthy. If you want to build a business, you'll be able to run on all cylinders. Your focus, motivation and energy will be one hundred percent! Want to spend more time with your kids being able to run and hike or go wake surfing at the lake? How about fitness? Want to turn heads this summer? No matter who you are. No matter how young or old you are, it's impossible to think about living a fulfilled life if you're not healthy. Now that we got that out of the way, let's talk about fasting.

Chapter 1. What Fasting Is

Fasting:
1.to abstain from all food
2.to eat only sparingly or of certain kinds of food

Fasting is voluntarily abstaining from eating. It's also known as time restricted eating. This implies there is a decision to eat or not eat. Starvation is involuntarily abstaining from food. Whether you want to eat or not, there is no choice. If you are starving, you have no way to eat nor do you know when your next meal is coming. In this chapter, we're going to introduce you to fasting and give you a basic understanding of how it works. Understanding this, you will give yourself a higher chance of making it work for you.

Let me be clear about one thing: Fasting is not for everyone. There are some people I would highly recommend DO NOT fast as it will backfire for you.

Who are these people?

•   Professional Athletes: Fasting is also not a wise choice for the professional athlete who is training multiple times per day. You NEED fuel to train with great intensity. Unless you are going for a brisk walk (which is completely fine to do while fasted), you need carbs and protein in your system. If you train in the morning, afternoon, and evening, then you need to eat throughout the entire day and fasting is not for you.

•   Children/Teens: Fasting is not a good idea for those under the age of 18. At this point in your life, you need an ongoing supply of good nutrition to support your growing body. Going for long periods without eating may hamper the natural growth that should occur during this time.

•   Type 2 Diabetics: Fasting is also not wise for those with type 2 diabetes. These individuals need an ongoing supply of snacks and meals in order to maintain proper blood glucose levels.

•   Pregnant/Nursing Women: The growing baby requires ongoing nutrition as well and lactating women who fast may see a severe decline in breast milk production.

•   Anemic Individuals: Those who suffer from anemia should avoid fasting as this may make their situation worse, as well as those who suffer from a rare condition called porphyria, in which chemical substances called porphyrins accumulate with high metabolism.

•   Those with a CoA deficiency: In this rare genetic condition, ketosis is prevented due to the fatty acid deficiency of acetyl-CoA. This means the body is not able to break down fats as a fuel source, thus making it very hard to fast for any length of time. In normal individuals, when circulating blood glucose and muscle glycogen (stored carbohydrates) are depleted, fatty acids then become the primary source of fuel and ketosis is established. Since this can't happen in those with CoA deficiency, they need to have a constant influx of glucose throughout the day to keep their brain and body fueled. Therefore, fasting is not an ideal option in this scenario.

Always consult your physician before starting any new diet or exercise plan.

WHO IS FASTING FOR?

Fasting is for those who:

•	Are tired of spending hours prepping and eating each day.

•	Have tried dieting but have been unsuccessful reaching their goals.

•	Want to get lean and stay lean all year long.

•	Live a busy life and don't want to stop to eat.

•	Are annoyed with eating small 'diet' meals and just want to eat satisfying meals.

•	Suffer from food cravings regularly and want to squash those.

•	Are looking to build muscle with the potential of losing fat at the same time.

•	Hope to enhance their insulin sensitivity and improve their health.

•	Are hoping to reduce their risk of illness and disease.

•	Want to control food, not have food control them.

In this book, you are going to learn the ins and outs of fasting. You are going to learn how to approach fasting, the best type of fasting to use for your personal goals and preferences, as well as how to implement controlled fasting successfully.

What will this book not be? This book will not be a plan that's going to hold your hand and tell you it's okay to eat what you want. There are specific ways of eating when fasting and you need to come to terms with realty: If you want to see great results, things need to change. If you are looking for a book that promises some easy to use secret that's virtually the same as what you are doing now but will lead to miraculous results, you are not going to find it here. I am not going to sugar coat anything. To truly change your body, it takes hard work and determination. Get that straight from day one and you will be off to a more successful start.

What I am going to provide you with here is a blueprint for leading your best life, should you choose to take it. I'm going to show you an alternative way of eating that has helped me attain the physique I have today, become far more productive with my time and learn to enjoy food a great deal more.

You will also be provided with the recipe for success if this is the path you want to take. I'm also going to show you some variations of fasting so that you can pick and choose which is the right method for you. No cookie-cutter approach here. You are looking for a way of eating and managing your diet that works with your body and your goals. Plain and simple. Customization is key.

This program can be used by both males and females, so there is no gender restriction here. Both young and old can do it. While I do recommend that you do not do this if you are under the age of 18 years and are still growing, anyone above that age who is interested can partake in a fasting approach. One side note: If you have a child who is overweight, please consult your physician and ask them if fasting is right for them.

Always speak to your doctor before adapting a new diet program however. I caution those who are suffering from diabetes about doing a fasting approach as it may impact your blood glucose levels in a negative manner. You'll want to speak with them first and discuss how you will handle that before moving forward.

Likewise, those with other serious medical conditions: heart disease, high blood pressure, and so on will also want to get their physician's clearance before proceeding with a fasting approach.

IS FASTING SAFE?

Right now, you might be wondering if fasting is safe? After all, it is planned starvation more or less—you are choosing not to eat. Is that really healthy?

For most of the population (go back and review the section for people who should not engage in fasting), it is a safe program. You aren't fasting for an extended period of time and are you are still taking in plenty of nutrient-dense foods each and every week (or you should be!).

Fasting over the long term—weeks, months, or longer is not a safe option but that's not what we're doing here each day. In fact, you'll still be taking in close to the same number of calories that you would on a diet if you weren't fasting on this approach, you're just changing the spacing of those calories out.

The body can go for long periods of time without food. Contrary to what you may have read, you do not need to be eating every 2-3 hours or your body will go into 'starvation' mode. Your body is equipped with very effective systems in place to ensure that you are prepared to manage longer periods without food. Not to worry—you are not going to starve to death by not eating for 12-22 hours a day.

What are some of the pros and cons of fasting?

The following are my opinions. Let's take a look.

PROS:

•   Increased time availability during the day (you aren't spending so much time meal prepping and eating!)

•   Improved hunger control

•   Enhanced blood glucose regulation

•   Improved insulin sensitivity

•   Enhanced weight loss results

•   Improved focused and clarity

•   Increased and stabilized energy levels

•   Enhanced longevity

- Faster metabolic rate

- Greater control over food intake

- Stronger immune system

- Potentially better skin and nail health

Cons:

- Some people may experience some hunger while they adapt to the plan

- Can be difficult to organize and attend social functions during the fasting window

- Potential to experience gastrointestinal upset due to eating a higher number of calories over a shorter timespan

- Females trying to become pregnant may notice changes in their reproductive system function and hormonal levels (always consult a physician before engaging in any diet program)

All in all, there aren't that many drawbacks to fasting and definitely not drawbacks that cannot be overcome, so this really is one type of protocol you will want to consider. We'll go more in detail on the pros and cons of fasting later on.

To further understand fasting and how it works, it's important to learn the basics of what happens in our body when we eat food.

Digestion

Digestion is a very complicated process and one that is quite amazing when you take a step back and look into it.

There are two phases of digestion to know: Mechanical digestion and chemical digestion. Let's take a look at mechanical digestion first.

Mechanical Digestion

Mechanical digestion occurs as soon as you put food into your mouth. Your teeth are designed to be able to break down the food into smaller bits, which will then make things easier for the rest of your digestive system in the chemical portion of digestion. It's also essential that you break the food down into smaller bits as this is what will allow it to pass through the throat without you choking.

Chemical Digestion

Chemical digestion is a lengthy process and begins as soon as you smell the food you are about to eat. Ever notice when you walk by a pizza shop in the mall and smell that aroma— your mouth starts watering?

Stage 1

Welcome to Stage 1 of digestion. The sensory stimulus of scent triggers our body to begin releasing saliva from the salivary glands, which contain a number of enzymes that are designed to break down the food that you just ate.

Some of the other main events that happen when you smell that delicious aroma of food include:

•	Stomach contractions (which are actually what people often feel as 'hunger pains')

•	Chemical release from the intestinal glands to prepare for the incoming food

STAGE 2

As you begin chewing the food, breaking it up, you'll then pass it down through the esophagus, which is a long tube that leads to your stomach. This tube has muscles that contract in wave-like motions to accomplish this task.

STAGE 3

Once the food reaches the stomach, the real work begins. Here, the stomach begins contracting forcefully, breaking the food down into extremely small pieces while stomach juices that have now been released begin the real chemical process of breaking the food down into proteins, carbohydrates, and fats. These stomach juices are made up of a blend of digestive enzymes, hydrochloric acid, and mucus.

STAGE 4

From here, the end product is a soupy concoction of the different macronutrients called chyme, and it begins to make its way to the small intestine for the absorption of those nutrients.

In the small intestine, there are a number of additional digestive juices that will help with absorption. This includes amylases which are secreted by the pancreas to help with carbohydrate digestion; bile from the liver and gallbladder to help to emulsify fats (mix it with water); and enzymes from the pancreas and intestine that will help with the separation of proteins and amino acids.

As the chyme moves into the intestines, it's absorbed through special cells in the walls that suck up all the sugars, amino acids, fatty acids, vitamins, and minerals. From here, they are then sent off to the respective places in the body where they are needed.

STAGE 5

In the second to last stage of digestion, whatever is left after all those important molecules that your body needs have been absorbed and is then left to move towards the large intestine and gets converted into feces, which is the waste that will then be removed. Any insoluble dietary fiber you ate is in this composition, which is not broken down by the body.

STAGE 6

This mixture passes through the large intestine, referred to as the colon, where any water in the mixture is absorbed. After this absorption, what's left is a very thick mixture, also known as feces (or poop), which is then passed out of the colon by way of strong large intestine muscles.

This completes the entire digestion process.

So, as you can see, digestion is definitely not a fast or simple process. Your body spends hours completing the digestion process—so much so, that for those on a typical 'eat every 3-4 hours' diet, you would still be digesting the previous meal while eating your current meal.

One of the beautiful things about the fasting approach is that you let your digestive system rest. You allow it to take a break when you are fasting to not be at work, which is part of the reason many report feeling so much more energized during their fast. They aren't weighed down by the constant digestion process that tends to occur.

IMPROVING THE DIGESTIVE SYSTEM

You might now wonder what you can do to improve your digestive processes? If you can enhance digestion and ensure it's functioning as best as possible, this is going to mean that you are able to better absorb the nutrients from your foods, better use those nutrients as energy, and become healthier overall.

There are a few ways you can go about doing this.

TAKING DIGESTIVE ENZYMES

In an ideal world, everyone would have everything they need to digest their food properly. Sadly, many people don't. Some do not produce enough of the digestive enzymes needed to break down the foods they eat, and others don't produce the enzyme at all. For instance, if you are severely lactose intolerant, you are not producing lactase, which digests the sugar found in milk.

You can help improve your digestive system by taking supplementary digestive enzymes, which will help fill the gaps in what your body is not making on its own.

USE A PROBIOTIC

The next way to improve digestion is to use a probiotic. Probiotics are live bacteria that live inside the gut and help with the digestive process. They also play a key role in immune health regulation, so they are important to consume for a variety of different reasons.

While most of us have some probiotics already living in our gut, we may not have optimal levels due to the types of foods we eat (not consuming sufficient levels of pre-biotics, which help the probiotics grow and multiply), too much stress, or the use of antibiotics.

Probiotics are also hugely helpful for helping those who suffer from IBS (irritable bowel syndrome) manage their symptoms, so that's yet another reason to be including them in your day. Everyone should be taking a good probiotic.

DECREASE YOUR EMOTIONAL STRESS

Another big issue that can halt digestion is too much emotional stress. When you are stressed, the hormonal environment in your body is going to change, putting you in a fight-or-flight scenario. When you are in this position, the sympathetic nervous system begins taking over. Digestion is part of the parasympathetic nervous system, so all that stress is essentially opposing the process of digestion, causing everything to run less efficiently.

If you ever feel your stomach tighten up into a ball of knots while you are stressed, just imagine how hard it is for any sort of digestion to take place after learning about the steps of digestion above.

Your body cannot continue to break down food and absorb those nutrients if you are that tense internally.

EAT MORE DIETARY FIBER

Adding more dietary fiber to your day is another great way to enhance digestion. Dietary fiber helps the food move more smoothly through the small intestine and the stomach, allowing it to be properly broken down and then moved to the large intestine to become waste.

Those who don't get enough dietary fiber often notice irregularity with their bowel movements, which is a sure-sign that their digestive system is not running smoothly.

You'll want to include both insoluble as well as soluble fiber in your diet. Insoluble fiber helps add bulk to your food intake and improves bowel formation while soluble dietary fiber helps with the absorption of water and prevents stools from becoming too watery.

Exercise Regularly

Exercising is also an important thing that you'll want to do if you hope to improve digestive health. Exercising regularly helps get your bowels moving, can assist with regularity, and keeps your organs in top shape.

Note: Don't exercise right after eating. If you do that, you're likely to experience cramping in the small intestine and stomach. Wait a good 1-2 hours after eating, if you can. This is another reason why I suggest working out in a fasted state.

Stay Hydrated

Finally, be sure that you stay hydrated. Dehydration can decrease the process of digestion because your body needs the water in order to properly break down the nutrients and absorb them into the body.

Drinking regularly throughout the day will help ensure that dehydration does not become a limiting problem for you. You will feel better and your workouts will be much more optimal.

If you follow these tips, you should notice that your digestive system moves along more smoothly and, as a result, you have better energy throughout the day.

TEF: The Thermic Effect of Food

Each and every time you eat food, regardless of what type of food it is, your body goes through this digestion process. As you saw above, there are a number of events that take place during digestion, thus, energy is going to be expended at this time. That energy is referred to as 'The Thermic Effect of Food', otherwise known as 'TEF' for short.

This represents how many calories you burn each day through the process of digestion alone.

So how does it stack up?

It depends on what you eat! Certain foods have a higher TEF value than other foods, so you can actually have some influence over this by adjusting and adapting your diet plan.

Proteins are the foods that contain the highest TEF value. Proteins are hard work for the body to break down, which is why you may often notice that you are feeling warm after eating a high protein meal. All that protein is causing your body to release a lot of energy as heat, thus your body temperature rises. For every 100 calories of pure protein you take in, your body is going to expend about 20-25 of those calories just breaking it down. This means you only net around 75-80 calories. While this 25-calorie burn may not seem like much, it does add up. If you eat 500 calories worth of protein each day, that's an additional 125 calories per day burned off and over a month's time, that's over a pound of body fat loss.

Carbohydrates and dietary fats don't have as high of a calorie burn due to TEF because they are more readily converted into energy in the body. Carbohydrates come in at around 4% TEF value while dietary fats are very efficient at 2% TEF value.

Dietary fiber is also not fully digested in the body, so that's something else to consider and why you often hear people talking about 'net' carb intake. This represents the total carbohydrates that a food has minus the fiber content. While soluble fiber actually has a net caloric value of around 2 calories per gram (rather than the 4 that is normally representative of carbohydrates), these individuals are not counting this in there. Note that insoluble fiber will be passed out of the body, so when you combine the two together, dietary fiber calories are exceptionally low.

The type of diet does influence your TEF value. If you are on a higher protein diet, which many people who are looking to lose fat choose, then you will burn off more calories during the day without changing anything else.

On a typical mixed diet, when calculating daily expenditures, the value of 10% for TEF is usually used; however, on a high protein diet, you may be able to bump this up closer to 15% due to that higher protein intake. You wouldn't use the full 20-25% because a large portion of the diet will still be carbohydrates and dietary fats—and because these values are lower, this means that it's going to bring that average number down.

Now that you understand more about the thermic effect of food, let's discuss another factor that plays a role in your progress and program: Insulin.

INSULIN

Insulin is a hormone in your body, made by the pancreas, that allows you to use sugar (glucose) from carbohydrates you eat and turn them into useable energy, or store it as glycogen for later use. Insulin is important because it is responsible for keeping your blood sugar levels stable. When you eat food, your blood sugar rises and your pancreas signals cells (called 'beta cells') to release insulin in your bloodstream to allow sugar to be converted to energy.

If your body has a tough time producing enough insulin, you can develop hyperglycemia (high blood sugar). If your beta cells in your pancreas are damaged or destroyed, your body won't be able to make insulin and you'll need insulin injections to avoid hyperglycemia. This is known as diabetes type I and II. Since our goal is improving health, we want to do what we can to improve insulin sensitivity (how responsive your cells are to insulin). Improving insulin sensitivity can help lower insulin resistance and the risk of hyperglycemia and diabetes. This can also help you burn more fat and build more muscle.

A long time ago, our society used to eat three square meals per day. Over time, the idea of adding more meals/snacks to our daily regimen has become very popular for many different kinds of people—ranging from average people trying to get in better shape to elite athletes and bodybuilders. This has both positive and negative effects depending on your goals. Bodybuilders are after building massive amounts of muscle, so this frequency of meals can prove beneficial due to the increased muscle protein synthesis it provides. However, these frequent meals (ranging upwards of 6-9 meals per day) keep insulin levels elevated. If insulin levels are elevated for extended periods of time, it can lead to insulin resistance and this is one of the reasons why people gain unwanted weight.

INSULIN RESISTANCE

Insulin resistance is one of the leading causes behind many diseases today. While it may only be the direct cause of one disease known today, diabetes, it is going to dramatically increase your risk of a number of different diseases. Insulin resistance is the cornerstone issue involved in metabolic syndrome X, which is a tri-factor condition involving insulin resistance, high triglycerides, and obesity. Together, when you suffer from all three, your risk of suffering from heart disease and/or heart attacks and strokes dramatically increases.

When you suffer from insulin resistance, your body is unable to process carbohydrates like it should. So, when you eat a higher carbohydrate meal, rather than insulin coming in and doing its job and moving the glucose to the muscle tissues for storage as muscle glycogen, the cells stop responding to insulin—or don't respond as well. So instead, the glucose just sits in the blood until eventually it gets converted into fat.

When this happens, you are going to develop plaque on your artery walls and if this plaque ever breaks off, platelets will now come in to repair the damage. The only problem is that now, because all this plaque is so built up, your arteries are now much narrower, so the platelets may actually block the artery entirely, preventing blood and oxygen from passing through. If this happens, a heart attack or a stroke is about to occur, depending on which blood vessel in the body it's happening to.

This is why watching your triglyceride levels and cholesterol, both of which are heavily influenced by the intake of sugar, is so critical.

There are many things that can be done to help reduce insulin resistance, including participating in a strength training program, getting enough sleep at night, as well as avoiding the consumption of processed foods and beverages.

In addition to that, we come to intermittent fasting. Research is showing that intermittent fasting is one of the best ways to increase insulin sensitivity and help turn this terrible sequence of events around in those who are suffering (Halberg et al. 2005).

This makes sense if you think about it from a logical perspective. When you are eating every few hours throughout the day, assuming those meals do contain some form of carbohydrate (and note even higher amounts of protein can increase insulin levels), you are keeping insulin constantly circulating around the blood. Over time, the cells adapt to this and they become less responsive. Why should they respond? High insulin becomes the norm—something that is typical and doesn't require a response.

When you fast however, there's no insulin being released because no food is coming in. Therefore, when your cells are finally met with insulin, they take action immediately because this powerful substance has a high influence over the cells responsible for the uptake of glucose.

What's more is that fasting may help accelerate fat loss progress as well. Whether you fast for 8-hours, 16-hours, or do a full 24-hour fast in an eat-stop-eat fashion, you are increasing the total amount of time during the day that the body is tapping into body fat stores (However, I do recommend you aim to fast for at least 16-hours because this is where the greatest advantages start to take place).

If you are eating every two-to-three hours, each time food comes in, your body goes from a catabolic (tissue breakdown) state to an anabolic (tissue building) one. While if you were trying to pack on 20 pounds of muscle mass, then this would probably be viewed as a good thing. During this time, you just have to accept that some body fat is going to be gained as a result of it.

When dieting however, you actually want to be in a catabolic state to some degree because this means the body is breaking down body fat tissue for energy. Basically, intermittent fasting is helping to elevate total adipose thermogenesis, as was shown by research published in the Cell Research journal (Kim et al. 2017).

This said, you want to avoid breaking down protein tissue as that means the loss of lean muscle mass, and you can avoid this by making sure that you are eating sufficient protein in your diet. When you have sufficient levels of protein coming in each day, your body is less likely to turn to lean tissue for use as an energy source and instead, turn almost fully towards body fat.

You can choose your length of fasting based on what you're comfortable with, but generally speaking, the longer you fast, the greater your insulin sensitivity will be. Fasting for 8-hours is very easy—just don't eat overnight while sleeping (which you likely already do) and then perhaps push breakfast by an hour or two, depending on how long you sleep and when you ate before bed.

If you want to fast for 12-hours, that's also not that difficult for most. Just skip eating right before bed and wait a few hours upon waking to eat breakfast.

Fasting for 16-hours? You'll avoid eating from 8pm until lunch the next day. This again is not actually all that hard. When you get busy in the morning, you'll find you forget to eat anyway and may appreciate not having to worry about preparing yourself breakfast any longer.

Fasting for 24-hours may be slightly more challenging, but I would recommend doing it from after dinner one night until that same time the next night. This way you aren't having to worry about going to bed hungry at any point in time. Those who fast for 24-hours typically alternate one day of fasting with one day of normal-style eating. Otherwise you're forced to try and get in a very high calorie intake in a very short eating timespan of about an hour, which can cause great gastrointestinal discomfort.

What is interesting is that research is showing one great advantage of the 24-hour fast and that is the development of beiging (Li et al. 2017). You may have never heard of this before, but essentially it is the stimulation of beige fat development within white adipose tissue that dramatically decreases obesity as well as insulin resistance. These findings all happen within the gut of the body and indicate that fat loss may have more to do with the simple energy-in versus energy-out model that has been preached for years and years. By implementing fasting every other day into your regime, you may actually create a shift in your physiology that changes how your body handles fat burning.

So, as you can see, as far as improving insulin sensitivity goes, intermittent fasting is one of the best things that you can possibly do. It's so good, in fact, that it may help to completely turn your health around, taking you from a high risk of heart disease to a much lower one.

If we eat meals regularly, our body metabolizes the food and turns it into usable energy, so we can do normal everyday things. But what happens when we fast?

How Fasting Works:

When you fast, your insulin levels drop because we aren't eating carbohydrates; there's no sugar for insulin to turn into usable energy or store as glycogen for later use. When we stop eating, our body still has to produce energy, so it begins a process called, 'gluconeogenesis'. Your body needs to produce sugar for energy, so your liver converts things like amino acids, fats, and lactate into glucose. This glucose will be used and converted into energy. Once that is depleted, it begins using stored body fat as fuel.

Just as insulin resistance can lead to unwanted weight gain, improved insulin sensitivity can lead to enhanced thermogenesis. When you fast, you are giving your body more time to do it's magic while insulin levels are low.

George Cahill, a leading fasting expert, describes the stages of fasting in more detail. Refer to Figure One. We will concentrate on a few of those stages here.

	I	II	III	IV	V
	0-4 hours	4-16 hours	16-32 hours	32 hrs to 24 d	24 days and on
Origin of blood glucose	Exogenous	Glycogen, Hepatic GNG	Hepatic GNG, glycogen	Hepatic and renal GNG	Hepatic and renal GNG
Tissues using glucose	All	All except liver. Muscle and adipose tissue of diminished rate	All except liver. Muscle and fat tissue at rates intermediary betw. II and IV	Brain, red blood cells, renal medulla. Small amount by muscle	Brain at a diminished rate, red blood cells, renal medulla
Major fuel of brain	Glucose	Glucose	Glucose	Glucose, ketone bodies	Ketone bodies, glucose

Figure One: The Stages of Fasting Physiology by George Cahill.

In The Fasting Plan, you won't be fasting for longer than 24-hours, so I want you to pay closer attention to what happens in your body during these first three stages.

STAGE ONE: HOURS 0-4 OF FASTING

You begin phase one of your fasting journey by having your last meal. During this first four-hours of time-restricted eating, your body is fueled primarily by exogenous sources of glucose. 'Exogenous sources' is a fancy way of saying we get this fuel from 'outside sources', meaning it's from the food we eat and not the glucose our body produces. The process of glycolysis (your body breaking down sugar into energy) takes place. During this phase, your hunger level is somewhat low, and your irritability level is tolerable. Most people have no problem getting through this phase.

STAGE TWO: HOURS 4-16 OF FASTING

Continuing our fasting journey, we proceed to phase two. This is the 4-16 hours after consuming your last meal. Glycogen fuel gets low and your body starts converting other sources into energy. The primary source of fuel here is hematic glycogen (glycogen stored in your liver). The body uses things like amino acids from protein, lactate, and glycerol and converts them into sugar to be used as fuel: This process is called 'gluconeogenesis'. The term literally translates to: "the making of (genesis) new (neo) sugar (glucose)". During this phase, hunger might creep in and you'll start to notice your stomach grumble. About half the people I've worked with say hunger is highest at this time and others say they are barely hungry at all. Opinions will vary, and you'll have to ride it out. (In the second half of the book where we discuss the application of the fasting plan, we'll go over some techniques and tips you can use to reduce or eliminate hunger altogether.)

STAGE THREE: HOURS 16-32 OF FASTING

Phase three of Cahill's fasting physiology takes place. This is the 16-32 hours after eating your last meal. Your body continues to convert hematic glycogen to fuel and produces its own energy (gluconeogenesis continues) and your stored glycogen levels are depleted. At this point, your body still needs fuel, so it turns to your stored fat and starts using them as energy (ketones). This is of course where the magic happens. As with anything, the toughest part of life often leads to the greatest rewards. Hunger levels will be the highest during this stage and irritability might follow. However, you may notice hunger coming and going many times. And the more you fast, the more comfortable you'll be. I truly believe it gets easier the more you use it.

Although the fasting plan won't have you fasting past stage 3 most of the time, it's worth covering stages 4 and 5 of Cahill's physiology of fasting so you'll have a basic understanding of fasting and what happens in our body when we fast for extended periods of time.

STAGES FOUR AND FIVE: HOURS 32+

Gluconeogenesis decreases significantly. Ketones become the major fuel for the brain. During these phases, you will start entering into ketosis. Ketosis is defined as "a metabolic state in which some of the body's energy supply comes from ketone bodies in the blood. Generally, ketosis occurs when the body is metabolizing fat at a high rate and converting fatty acids into ketones."

AUTOPHAGY

In addition to all these great benefits, there's one other additional magical thing that happens when you fast for an extended period of time: Autophagy. Autophagy is basically the self-destruction of your own body. Sounds scary, right? Don't be scared. It's actually a good thing. When you fast for an extended period of time, your body will begin essentially eating itself, but the good news is that the cells and tissues it chooses to eat are actually ones that you want to do away with anyway. Think of this as your body's own natural recycling program, where it takes out the waste and makes room for better, stronger tissues. If you fast long enough, you turn on this recycling program and make great strides in your health.

As you progress through the fast, the body is going to begin eating up scraps of dead, diseased, and worn-out cells, all of which could lead you down a path to cancer, diabetes, and metabolic dysfunction (Coupé et al. 2012). These harmful cells are eaten up and used for further energy to help boost the immune system and improve overall functionality. In fact, autophagy may also help boost brain health, reducing the risk of Alzheimer's disease or Parkinson's disease.

THE CIRCADIAN RHYTHM

Until recently, humans have always eaten during the day and fasted during the night. Back in the day, there was nothing to do at night but read or talk to their partner. That can only keep you occupied for so many hours, right? With the recent invention of electricity in the recent years, we now have the opportunity to do anything we want at any time of the day. While this gives us options to freely do as we please, it isn't necessarily good for our circadian rhythm. Our circadian rhythm is our own internal clock that regulates our natural inclinations to eat, sleep, and feel active during the day. Our circadian rhythm is also responsible for other hormone functions like testosterone production and the release of cortisol (our stress hormone).

Think about this: Now we have longer days (more light) so we stay up longer. It is natural for us to have the desire to eat while we are up, so more food is eaten. Not only this, we end up waking up at the same time; so we stay up longer, eat more food, and sleep less because our circadian rhythm is out of whack. By restricting the times you eat, you might be able to see how intermittent fasting may help you improve your feeding patterns and restore your circadian rhythm.

Is Fasting Difficult?

Many people avoid fasting because they think it's going to be too hard! You might feel your stomach growl after an hour of not eating and think to yourself, "How could I ever go 16-hours without eating?" NEVER!

Well, it's not as hard as it seems. Sure, the first day or two that you do it, you might find it a bit challenging. But beyond that, it gets so much easier. The human body is highly adaptable and the longer you fast, the more your body learns that this is the new norm—the new way of eating and hunger adjusts with it. In fact, many people have to remind themselves to break the fast and start eating again.

When fasting, your body is going to be releasing endorphins, which serve to both energize you (one of the many great benefits of fasting) and help to squash hunger. You'll feel clear minded, light, and not weighed down like you may have previously.

Remember back when you first switched over to a six-meal per day protocol? Perhaps you first started your health kick and went from eating three main meals a day to eating six smaller meals. How did you feel? Most people report feeling stuffed! They can't eat so often, they just aren't hungry. But if you stuck it out and kept forcing yourself to eat, soon you became hungry. Your body learned to expect food at these times and it was just normal to you.

The same happens when you begin intermittent fasting, just in reverse. It can take a bit of time to adapt but once you do, you won't think twice about it. Remember that we all have pounds and pounds of fat stores, equating to thousands of calories at our disposal. Your body has zero risk of starving to death unless you are one of the very few people in the bodybuilding culture that has low, single-digit levels of body fat.

KETOSIS AND FASTING

Another thing to keep in mind is that if you are someone who is interested in going on the ketogenic diet, fasting is actually one of the best ways to utilize this approach. In the ketogenic diet, your goal is to deprive the body of glucose in order to get it into a state of ketosis faster, which then forces the body to run on an alternative source of fuel called 'ketone bodies'. These ketone bodies help keep blood glucose very stable and assist with overall rates of fat burning.

Essentially intermittent fasting and ketogenic diets have very similar goals, the big difference is ketogenic diets prescribe the macronutrient ratio to follow while intermittent fasting prescribes the eating schedule to follow.

For those doing ketogenic diets, using intermittent fasting to quickly get into ketosis can greatly assist your progress. What better way to get your body using ketones a fuel source than to completely deprive it from all food together?

Often the hardest thing about using a ketogenic diet is that initial period where you have to adapt and get into ketosis, and intermittent fasting can be the single best way to speed this process along.

Understand: Our bodies are incredibly adaptive and it's perfectly natural to fast, allowing us to use our stored fuel more efficiently. Insulin will rise when we eat and fall when we fast. Consistently lowering insulin levels can lead to improved insulin sensitivity. If we can improve insulin sensitivity, our body improves its ability to build muscle and burn fat. Not only this, lower insulin can help you rid your body of excess water and salt. Muscle building, fat burning, and an overall lighter feeling of becoming a lean, mean machine? I told you this stuff was cool.

Now you have a basic understanding of what happens in your body when you engage in a period of time-restricted eating.

If you're interested in learning more about fasting and how it can benefit your health, body, and mind, continue reading to find out... "Why Fasting Is Awesome".

CHAPTER 1 KEY TAKEAWAYS:

•   Fasting: choosing to eat little or no food for a certain time period. Also known as 'time-restricted eating'. Don't confuse it with starvation.

•   Challenge your way of thinking by learning and applying the principles of fasting and never stop questioning the validity of any program.

•   When you eat, insulin rises by turning food into energy.

•   Unhealthy insulin levels can lead to disease like type I and II diabetes.

•   When you fast, your insulin levels drop. This can help improve insulin sensitivity. Improved insulin sensitivity can help your body become more effective at burning fat and building muscle.

CHAPTER REFERENCES

Halberg, N., Henriksen, M., Söderhamn, N., Stallknecht, B., Ploug, T., Schjerling, P., & Dela, F. (2005, December). Effect of intermittent fasting and refeeding on insulin action in healthy men. Retrieved from https://www.ncbi.nlm.nih.gov/pubmed/16051710

Kim, K. H., Kim, Y. H., Son, J. E., Lee, J. H., Kim, S., Choe, M. S., . . . Sung, H. K. (2017, November). Intermittent fasting promotes adipose thermogenesis and metabolic homeostasis via VEGF-mediated alternative activation of macrophage. Retrieved from https://www.ncbi.nlm.nih.gov/pubmed/29039412

Li, G., Xie, C., Lu, S., Nichols, R. G., Tian, Y., Li, L., . . . Gonzales, F. J. (2017, October). Intermittent fasting promotes white adipose browning and decreases obesity by shaping the gut microbiota. Retrieved from https://www.cell.com/cell-metabolism/fulltext/S1550-4131(17)30504-1

Coupé, B., Ishii, Y., Dietrich, M. O., Komatsu, M., Horvath, T. L., & Bouret, S. G. (2012, February 08). Loss of autophagy in pro-opiomelanocortin neurons perturbs axon growth and causes metabolic dysregulation. Retrieved from https://www.ncbi.nlm.nih.gov/pubmed/22285542

Chapter 2: Why Fasting Is Awesome

"Fasting is the first principle of medicine; fast and see the
strength of the spirit reveal itself."
-Rumi

Fasting is awesome. Period. It's been around for a hell of a long time and people continue to talk about it because it works. It's good for your health, body, and mind. The goal of this chapter is to convince you it is as awesome as I think it is. No matter what health goal you're aiming towards, the benefits of fasting are too good to be ignored.

How old are you? After you answer that question to yourself, think about this. If you've never fasted before, there's a decent chance you've gone your entire life eating breakfast, lunch and dinner. This means your digestive system has received a break exactly ZERO times. No matter what age you are, that is a heck of a long time to go without giving your body a chance to rest. Think of your body like RAM on a computer. Each computer has a certain amount of random access memory (RAM). The RAM allows the computer to run different programs simultaneously and efficiently. If your computer is dedicating the majority of its RAM towards one program, the other programs begin to suffer and the whole computer starts to slow down. Once you figure out which program is taking up all the RAM, you can shut it down and— voila! The computer starts to run optimally again! Your body is the same way. By giving your digestive system a break, it can devote its resources towards detoxification and autophagy (cell-cleansing), disease prevention, thermogenesis, improved insulin sensitivity, and more things that make you healthy, fit, and strong.

Fasting has been getting a lot of attention in the media for the last few years due to its tremendous health benefits. In this chapter, we are going to cover many of the positive benefits by discussing what the studies are showing. It is our goal to provide you with a better framework and understanding of why you might be able to use intermittent fasting as a conduit to improve your general health and increase your fat-burning capabilities.

In this book, we are mainly focused on fat-burning, so we will break down studies as it relates to fat-burning in particular.

IMPROVING YOUR HEALTH, ONE DAY AT A TIME

It's important that you are constantly taking steps to improve your health. Even if you aren't in a disease-ridden state, you still must be taking measures to help prevent diseases from occurring. Otherwise, you will end up reacting instead of preventing. The good news is fasting can significantly improve your general health.

FASTING ASSISTS WITH CELL REPAIR AND REGENERATION

Each and every day, your cells are constantly turning over and remodeling. They're breaking down, re-growing, and (hopefully) making you stronger. If the body slows down at the process of regeneration of the cells, this is when old and worn out cells that aren't doing their job properly begin to reign over and health problems set in. A rapid rate of regeneration therefore is critical to sustaining optimal health.

When you fast, a process called neuronal autophagy is enhanced, which is the key process where cytosolic components are degraded and recycled through lysosomes—where new cells are created.

As was stated in one study published in the Autophagy journal, "one well-recognized way of inducing autophagy is by food restriction, which up regulates autophagy in many organs including the liver" (Alirezai et al. 2010). The study goes on to point out that autophagy has been recognized as a crucial defense mechanism to protect against malignancy (cancer), infection, Alzheimer's disease, and neurodegenerative diseases.

FASTING MIGHT COMBAT AGING

Want to find a way to turn back the hands of time? While you may not be able to completely reverse aging, the good news is that you may be able to slow it down. Research has now illustrated that intermittent fasting appears to be a fantastic way to prevent the cellular decay process and help protect your body against diseases along with the wear and tear that comes with the process of getting older.

In a recent study published in 2018 in the journal Molecular Cell, fasting was shown to produce a molecule that delays vascular aging. In this study, researchers looked at the link between calorie restriction and vascular aging in mice. They induced starvation and the rodents produced the molecule beta-hydroxbutyrate, a ketone created by the liver in the absence of glucose. Now, here is the cool part. The findings indicated that Beta-hydroxbutyrate promotes amitosis (cell division) inside of blood vessels. And this is a marker of cellular youth (Han, 2018).

Many people, when thinking about the aging process, tend to mostly think about getting wrinkles and losing muscle mass tissue, but it's so much more than this. The biggest part of aging takes place on the inside, which you can't see, but will definitely be impacted. If you aren't careful in taking preventative measures, you will may wind up in serious health trouble.

Some scientists have gone so far as to claim that fasting may help to cut the risk of cancer and diabetes by half, two of the biggest diseases taking lives everywhere (Knapton, 2015).

Some of the greatest risk factors for aging include fat distribution, blood pressure, and levels of insulin-like growth factor (IGF-1). A study published in the Science Translational Medicine journal noted that patients performing a 'fasting mimicking diet' (FMD) five-consecutive days per month for a three-month timespan improved all of these ratings and put subjects at a reduced risk of experiencing age-related diseases (Wei et al. 2017). The FMD involves a very low-calorie approach rather than complete fasting, but it's carried out for five days. On day one, just over 1000 calories are consumed and on days two to five, 725 calories are eaten. Because the food intake is so low, it's been said it can provide similar benefits to fasting.

There's no question however that whether you choose this approach or an intermittent fasting approach where you go completely without food for a set period of time, you will be reaping anti-aging benefits.

Fasting Might Improve Cardiovascular Health

Fasting can lead to improved cardiovascular health and there are three possible explanations. First, as shown by research, individuals who fast regularly have better self-control. I believe this is because folks learn to identify with true hunger compared to emotional hunger. This leads to healthier eating choices and ultimately helps them to consume fewer calories, even when they aren't fasting.

The second reason could be the changes in the way body metabolizes cholesterol in the fasting periods. When you fast, your body decreases its content of LDL (Low Density Lipoprotein or 'bad cholesterol') and increases the content of HDL (High Density Lipoprotein or 'good cholesterol').

Finally, fasting fine-tunes your body's ability to metabolize blood sugar. This way, fasting controls your cholesterol levels and improves blood sugar levels—both of which are directly linked to your cardiovascular well-being (Collier, 2013).

Fasting Boosts the Immune System

It is a well-known fact that a healthy lifestyle boosts the immune system. And what could be a better way to do it than fasting. Researchers have studied the effects of the functioning of the immune system in individuals with Multiple Sclerosis (MS). MS is an autoimmune condition characterized by the immune destruction of myelin—the protective covering surrounding the neurons. The benefits of fasting in such conditions include improvement in the levels of corticosterone, which helps reduce the levels of inflammation and abnormal immune activation. Fasting also helps reduce the levels of a variety of T helper cells (Th cells) and Antigen Presenting Cells (APCs). These cells serve as the precursor cells for promoting autoimmunity.

Fasting helps reduce the measure of pro-inflammatory chemicals called cytokines. Increased levels of these chemicals also cause aberrant immune activation. Also, fasting not only helps prevent the worsening of MS symptoms by suppressing immunity but helps reverse the symptoms as well by triggering the regeneration of myelin sheath (Choi et al. 2016).

Fasting Enhances Mental Health

Want to give your brain a boost? Research has demonstrated that fasting may help to improve brain health by increasing the synaptic plasticity of the brain, improving performance of memory tests and help promote the growth of new neurons. It may also help to enhance recovery after stroke or traumatic brain injury while decreasing the risk for neurodegenerative diseases like Alzheimer's and Parkinson's disease (Bair, 2015).

This research provides promising hope for the aging population who is at a higher risk for experiencing downward turns to their mental health and who may use intermittent fasting as a means of helping to boost their brain power.

Some people have also reported that intermittent fasting may help to treat mood related disorders such as anxiety and depression. It's far better to resort to natural alternative remedies than relying on medications for these conditions, so restructuring your eating pattern is a great way to achieve this.

FASTING IMPROVES METABOLISM

Fasting regulates digestion and helps in promoting healthy bowel functioning. There is also research showing that intermittent fasting promotes resting energy expenditure and boosts metabolism (Reinersen & Haftorn, 1984). The body also releases HGH (Human Growth Hormone) which helps in burning excessive body fat and maintaining body muscle.

Fasting cleans your internal organs and can help you get rid of the excess toxins. Because of all this, it becomes very clear that fasting can be an excellent way to help lose weight and burn off excess body fat. In addition to helping to improve the overall metabolic rate as noted above, fasting also helps out in a few other ways.

It helps increases insulin sensitivity (Patterson et al. 2015). The more sensitive your body is to glucose, the better it will be able to direct incoming glucose to the muscle tissues for storage as muscle glycogen and the less likely it will be to shuttle that glucose off to body fat storage instead. Most people who are currently overweight and eating a diet rich in processed foods have incredibly poor insulin sensitivity, which is in part why we see the rates of obesity and diabetes we do today.

Fasting may also help you enter a state called ketosis. You've probably heard about ketosis before, and for good reason. It's become a very popular weight loss strategy. If you are in good physical condition and are eating a healthy diet, your body does a good job turning calories into usable energy and doesn't normally make ketones. If your diet doesn't provide you with enough carbohydrates, your body can switch to ketosis and burn fat for energy instead. In this state, your body stops running off glucose as a fuel source and starts using ketone bodies. (Dashti et al. 2004). When this takes place, blood glucose levels are extremely well stabilized and energy levels are kept very constant. The biggest benefit however is that, in ketosis, appetite nearly ceases to exist, so this makes it very easy to control your food intake.

Many people are tentative about starting an intermittent fasting diet because they fear being hungry all day long since they can't eat for so many hours but typically, once the body is adapted, the opposite occurs. They need to remind themselves to eat when it's time to break the fast at the end of the day. If you have no appetite to eat, it becomes that much easier to control the calories in part of the weight loss equation.

Finally, fasting may also help with improving hormone sensitive lipase. This is an enzyme that is produced in the body to help release the fatty acids from the fat cells, which then provides energy to use during fat burning. Think of this enzyme as the direct controller over whether you are currently in a fat burning state or not. When hormone sensitive lipase is high, fat burning is taking place at an accelerated rate. When hormone sensitive lipase is not being released, no fat burning is occurring. What directly controls the release of hormone sensitive lipase?

Insulin. Whenever insulin is present, such as after a meal, especially one containing carbohydrates, it essentially puts the breaks on this enzyme. That means, you move out of a state of fat burning. By doing intermittent fasting, you help this enzyme become more predominant throughout the day, giving you more overall time in the fat burning state.

There's nothing magical about intermittent fasting that means you can eat anything and everything and still lose fat. It still comes down to the total amount of calories you eat. To burn fat, you still need to create a calorie restriction (I'll discuss this in detail in chapter 5: The Basics of Nutrition). However, the amazing thing about intermittent fasting is that it trains your body and mind to be more optimal and efficient. This will give you more control over your life. And guess what? This will ultimately leave you with a leaner, more chiseled physique. Pretty rad, right?

CHAPTER 2 KEY TAKEAWAYS

• Fasting gives your digestive system a break so it can devote its resources towards detoxification and autophagy, disease prevention, thermogenesis, improved insulin sensitivity, and more things that make you healthy, fit, and strong.

•   When you fast, a metabolic process called autophagy begins. Autophagy has been recognized as a crucial defense mechanism to protect against malignancy (cancer), infection, Alzheimer's disease, and neurodegenerative diseases.

•   Fasting may serve as a tremendous preventative measure against aging. Fasting can serve as a very effective preventative measure to combat the sings of aging and should be taken advantage of.

•   If you're trying to improve your cardiovascular health, fasting can help in the following ways.

1)   It will help you with self-control.

2)   Your body metabolizes cholesterol when you fast by decreasing the content of LDL levels and increases your HDL levels.

3)   Fasting fine-tunes your body's ability to metabolize blood sugar.

•   Fasting boosts the immune system by improving levels of corticosterone, which helps reduce the levels of inflammation and abnormal immune activation.

•   Fasting may help to improve brain health by increasing the synaptic plasticity of the brain.

•   There is new research showing that fasting is improving metabolism and insulin sensitivity. When you fast, you also release your body's HGH, which will help you get lean and stay lean.

Chapter References

Lennox, W. G., & Cobb, S. (1928, October). Studies in epilepsy viii. the clinical effects of fasting. Retrieved from https://jamanetwork.com/journals/archneurpsyc/article-abstract/644088

Navarro, S., Ros, E., Aused, R., García Pugés, A. M., Piqué, J. M., & Bonet, J. V. (1984). Comparison of fasting, nasogastric suction and cimetidine in the treatment of acute pancreatitis. Retrieved from https://www.karger.com/Article/Abstract/199112

Alirezai, M., Kemball, C. C., Flynn, C. T., Wood, M. R., Whitton, J. L., & Kiosses, W.B. (2010, August). Short-term fasting induces profound neuronal autophagy. Retrieved from https://www.ncbi.nlm.nih.gov/pmc/articles/PMC3106288/

Wei, M., Brandhorst, S., Shelehchi, M., Mirzaei, H., Cheng, C. W., Budniak, J., . . . Longo, V.D. (2017, February). Fasting-mimicking diet and markers/risk factors for aging, diabetes, cancer, and cardiovascular disease. Retrieved from https://www.ncbi.nlm.nih.gov/pubmed/28202779

Knapton, S. (2015, June). The fasting mimicking diet (fmd) improves longevity while cutting the risk of cancer and diabetes by half, scientists have found. Retrieved from https://www.telegraph.co.uk/science/2018/03/27/five-day-fasting-diet-slows-ageing-may-add-years-life/

Collier, R. (2013, June). Intermittent fasting: the science of going without. Retrieved from https://www.ncbi.nlm.nih.gov/pmc/articles/PMC3680567/

Choi, I. Y., Piccio, L., Childress, P., Bollman, B., Ghosh, A., Brandhorst, S., . . . Longo, V. D. (2016, May). Diet mimicking fasting promotes regeneration and reduces autoimmunity and multiple sclerosis symptoms. Retrieved from https://www.ncbi.nlm.nih.gov/pmc/articles/PMC4899145/

Wegman, M. P., Guo, M. H., Bennion, D. M., Shankar M. N., Chrzanowski, S. M., & Goldberg, L. A. (2015, April). Practicality of intermittent fasting in humans and its effect on oxidative stress and genes related to aging and metabolism. Retrieved from https://www.ncbi.nlm.nih.gov/pubmed/25546413

Hayati, F., Maleki, M., Pourmohommad, M., Sardari, K., Mohri, M., & Afkhami, A. (2011, February). Influence of Short-term, Repeated fasting on the skin wound healing of female mice. Retrieved from https://www.ncbi.nlm.nih.gov/pubmed/25881054

Bair, S. (2015, January). Intermittent fasting: try this at home for brain health. Retrieved from https://law.stanford.edu/2015/01/09/lawandbiosciences-2015-01-09-intermittent-fasting-try-this-at-home-for-brain-health/

Reinersen, R. E., & Haftorn, S. (1984, January). The effect of short-time fasting on metabolism and nocturnal hypothermia in the willow titparus montanus. Retrieved from https://link.springer.com/article/10.1007/BF00683212

Patterson, R. E., Laughlin, G. A., Sears, D. D., LaCroix, A. Z., Marinac, C., Gallo, L. C., . . . Villaseñor, A. (2015, April). Intermittent fasting and human metabolic health. Retrieved from https://www.ncbi.nlm.nih.gov/pmc/articles/PMC4516560/

Dashti, H. M., Mathew, T. C., Hussein, T., Asfar, S. K., Behbahani, A., Khoursheed, M. A., . . . Al-Zaid, N. S. (2004). Long-term effects of a ketogenic diet in obese patients. Retrieved from https://www.ncbi.nlm.nih.gov/pmc/articles/PMC2716748/

Ho, K. Y., Velduis, J. D., Johnson, M. L., Furlanetto, R., Evans, W. S., Alberti, K. G., & Thorner, M. O. (1988, April). Fasting enhances growth hormone secretion and amplifies the complex rhythms of growth hormone secrete in man. Retrieved from https://www.ncbi.nlm.nih.gov/pmc/articles/PMC329619/

Blackman, M. R., Sorkin, J. D., Münzer, T., Bellantoni, M. F., Busby-Whitehead, J., Stevens, T. E., . . . Harman, S. M. (2002, November). Growth hormone and sex steroid administration in healthy aged women and men: a randomized controlled trial. Retrieved from https://www.ncbi.nlm.nih.gov/pubmed/12425705

Li, L., Wang, Z., & Zuo, Z. (2013). Chronic intermittent fasting improves cognitive functions and brain structures in mice. Retrieved from https://www.ncbi.nlm.nih.gov/pmc/articles/PMC3670843/

Moro, T., Tinsley, G., Bianco, A., Marcolin, G., Pacelli, Q. F., Battaglia, G., . . . Paoli, A. (2016, October). Effects of eight weeks of time-restricted feeding (16/8) on basal metabolism, maximal strength, body composition, inflammation, and cardiovascular risk factors in resistance-trained males. Retrieved from https://www.ncbi.nlm.nih.gov/pmc/articles/PMC5064803/

Khamsi, R. (2006, October). Fasting may boost recovery from spinal injury. Retrieved from https://www.newscientist.com/article/dn10386-fasting-may-boost-recovery-from-spinal-injury/

Han, Y., Bedarida, T., Ding, Y., Somba, B. K., Lu, Q., Wang, Q., ... Zou, M.-H. (2018). β-Hydroxybutyrate Prevents Vascular Senescence through hnRNP A1-Mediated Upregulation of Oct4. Molecular Cell.

CHAPTER 3: FASTING MYTHS

"There are things known and there are things unknown, and
in between are the doors of perception."
-Aldous Huxley

Throughout our lives, we are faced with rumors, perceptions, and understandings of different ideas. If we believe these perceptions to be truths, that is what they are. If we decide to have an open mind, we unconsciously give ourselves a new way of looking at an event or situation and actively assess new information as it is presented to us in a fair way. This is really what allows us to improve. As human beings, it is in our nature to continue seeking the truth in all things. In my opinion, this is why it's so fun to find out if a myth is true or not. Shows like 'Myth Busters' are living proof of our interest in myths.

Fasting is one of those subjects that happens to include numerous myths. Before I actually did my own research on the subject, I thought many of the myths we'll cover were actually true.

In this chapter, we're going to break down these infamous myths and put them to rest for good. It is my belief that once you really understand the truth behind fasting, you'll be able to put one hundred percent confidence into it. And guess, what? Believing in something and knowing more about it can and will help you make it work for you.

Let's get to it.

MYTH #1: FASTING WILL MAKE YOU LOSE MUSCLE.

If I don't eat, I'll wither away and look like someone who's dying of starvation, right? What about the bodybuilders who preach eating every 3-hours of the day to make sure they don't lose muscle? Yeah, I wondered the same things to myself before I experimented with fasting.

Here is the reality. Fasting is voluntarily abstaining for food for a limited amount of time. It's not the same thing as starving. If you're starving, you're going to lose muscle of course. If you're fasting, you're simply going through a phase of time-restricted eating followed by a feeding window.

This myth really has nothing to do with fasting. It depends solely on calories in and calories out. The basic physiology of how our body's gain/lose weight is simple. If you eat more food than your body burns/uses, you will gain weight. If you eat less food than your body burns/uses, you'll lose weight.

Want to build muscle? Make sure you get enough calories in each day to support it. This means that you need to consume a surplus of calories during your feeding window, so you can support the muscle you are trying to build. This will be covered more in 'Chapter 6: The Basics: What you need to know about fasting'.

MYTH #2: FASTING IS UNHEALTHY.

If you're reading this now, you've read 'Chapter 2: Why Fasting Is Awesome', so you know fasting is extremely healthy. There are many different links to studies to show why fasting might benefit you and your health.

Fasting gives your digestive system a break so your body can focus more on amazing things like autophagy, thermogenesis, hypertrophy, and disease prevention. If you're still curious about the benefits of fasting, I've included a few authorities on the subject of time-restricted eating in the 'Resources' section in the back of the book.

MYTH #3: DOES FASTING DEPRIVE YOUR BODY OF ESSENTIAL NUTRIENTS?

When you fast, the first thing your body uses for energy is carbs and when the supply of carbs runs dry, it moves onto burning fat. People believe that when the body runs out of carbs, it starts to nibble away at proteins. This is NOT true at all!

First thing you need to note is that your body needs two types of nutrients: macronutrients (proteins, carbohydrates, and fats) and micronutrients (minerals and vitamins).

Let's talk about macronutrients first. These are easily available in food and at the same time are easy for the body to store. The carbohydrates are the first nutrient that our body breaks down to get energy. We all love carbs because this group includes cakes, bread, pasta, and cookies.

Fats are stored in our body as an energy reserve. The proteins that we consume are used to perform various functions in our body and build up muscles. Carbohydrates are not essential for the body; while proteins (amino acids) and fats (essential fatty acids) are.

When you fast, the fats burn to power your body. However, this does not include the essential fatty acids as they are stored and not used for the generation of energy. In addition, the old proteins breakdown into amino acids and build new proteins. This does not, in any way, affect the muscle mass.

Now, let's have a look at micronutrients. These nutrients include vitamins and minerals. Minerals like calcium, magnesium, and phosphorous are stored in the bones. That is why fasting does not have any significant impact on minerals in the body. Vitamins are fat soluble (vitamin A, D, E and K) and water soluble (vitamin B and C). The water-soluble vitamins are hard to store while the fat-soluble vitamins are stored in fat and your body maintains a good reserve of them.

Your body is very efficient and it's good at storing reserves of nutrients. When you employ The Fasting Plan, you actually give your body a chance to focus its resources on cool things like cell-cleansing (autophagy), thermogenesis, and hypertrophy instead of digestion. Fasting a day or two won't rob your body of nutrients. The food we eat after we break our fast is generally enough to fulfil our nutrient requirements.

The nutrients you get in your diet have more to do with the quality and selection of foods you consume. So, choose nutrient-dense foods to break your fast and you'll feel the results. This being said, it's pretty tough to get every single nutrient you need in the foods you consume. For this reason, I take a multivitamin.

MYTH #4: INTERMITTENT FASTING MAKES YOU LOSE MUSCLE.

Weight has been a concern of the human species since the ancient times. In the past, exercise methods and strict diets were no less than torture. People freaking hate diets, right?

Let's clear one thing, weight gain and weight loss are dietary problems and you can't simply exercise your way out of it.

So, the question is: Does fasting burn muscles? The simple answer is: NO!

Now, let's look at a little evidence to support this answer. Here we will discuss Dr. Kevin Hall's book 'Comparative Physiology of Fasting, Starvation and Food Limitation'.

In his book, Dr. Hall said that at the initial stage of fasting our body burns carbs (sugar) and when the carb storage run dry, the body turns to fat. Guess what? Whether you fast or not, you still have to understand the principle I mentioned above.

Eat more than your body uses = gain weight.

Eat less than your body uses = lose weight.

One of the reasons I believe fasting works so well is that it naturally teaches you to auto regulate your appetite. This means you'll learn to eat when you actually NEED to eat instead of just eating for the sake of eating. Fasting during the day and feasting in the evening is much easier to stick to and will give you a much better chance to create a calorie deficit needed to burn fat.

All we are really doing is changing the times we eat, not what we eat (for the most part). Simply put, you can stop worrying about losing muscle with intermittent fasting and start focusing on LIVING a kick-ass healthy life doing what you love.

MYTH #5: INTERMITTENT FASTING MAKES YOU OVEREAT.

Let's think logically on this one.

Normally, a person eats breakfast, lunch, and dinner and even includes some snacks here and there. In this example, let's say you start your day between 6 am and finish around 6 pm. Your day breaks out like this:

7 am: Eat breakfast of eggs, toast, and orange juice.

7:30 am: Order a Starbucks cinnamon dulce at the drive-through on your way to work.

10:30 am: At work, you grab a bagel with cream cheese from the break room.

12:30 pm: You go out to lunch with your co-workers, order a Caesar salad, and wash it down with a Diet Coke.

3:00 pm: Have a few handfuls of the trail mix you have hidden in your desk drawer at work.

6:00 pm: You get home from work and it's dinner time...

During that 12-hours, that's a hell of a lot of calories to consume. If we're not careful, it all adds up fast and, before we know it, we've created a surplus of calories that will probably go to fat storage. For most people, I've found this amount of calories consumed during the day is approximately 2,000 calories and higher. Remember, if you eat more calories than your body uses, you'll gain weight. If you eat less calories than your body uses, you'll lose weight. They say the average person needs around 2,000 calories to stay the same weight (maintenance calories). In this example, you've already ate your maintenance calories before you even get to eat dinner! That sucks, right?

Logically, fasting is amazing right off the bat because it gives you this extra cushion of time! If you like food like me, it's easy to overeat during the day. Instead of worrying about constricting calories and counting everything you eat, try changing the times you eat. Let's use another example involving controlled fasting.

6:00 am: You wake up and drink 24 oz of water.

7:30 am: Order a Starbucks drip coffee with trace amounts of cream at the drive-through on your way to work.

2:00 pm: You have a small plate of veggies with hummus to curb your hunger.

6:00 pm: You get home from work and it's dinner time...

In this example, you've created a cushion for yourself with your calories. You now have the rest of the night to eat. Eating 2,000 calories is quite a bit of food to consume in one meal, especially if it's from nutrient-dense sources.

In this myth, some say fasting causes you to overeat. Nope. EATING is what makes you overeat. Not fasting.

MYTH #6: FASTING WILL MAKE YOU LOSE ENERGY.

Many people often think that fasting will cause a significant decline in energy. After all, you aren't eating—so without fuel, surely you're going to be hungry, right? Not necessarily.

Here's the thing to remember. First, your body doesn't work on an hour by hour scale. In fact, it can take hours for you to digest your last meal. So as long as you are getting in the right number of total calories per day, your body still has the energy reserves.

Second, most people actually report feeling more energized, not less while fasting. This is because when you fast, your body is going to kick out endorphins as part of the process.

Think back to the hunter and gatherer days as this is what our bodies have evolved from.

When food was not available, what would happen? The men would have to go out and hunt it down—an energy consuming process for sure. They needed the energy to chase after these animals, thus their body evolved a way to deliver it: Adrenaline1.

Most of you have already heard about or know what adrenaline is. It's essentially a hormone that floods your system whenever you are doing something that awakens your body. If you sky-dive for instance, most people will say they get a great kick of adrenaline. It's something that happens when you do something exhilarating and it dramatically ups your energy level.

Fasting causes it to be released as well, so you can rest assured that low energy is not something you are likely to suffer from when fasting. If anything, you may notice your energy level goes up. This is one reason that many people actually keep going about their fasting program—they find it helps boost their energy so much during the day.

As many of you know, eating can actually cause your energy level to drop. When you eat, your parasympathetic nervous system kicks in, which is the system that is designed for 'rest and digest'. Ever notice how after lunch, you always want to take a mid-day nap? That's this concept at work.

So, by fasting, you focus more without the parasympathetic nervous system all day long, which keeps you energized and productive.

MYTH #7: FASTING CAUSES HYPOGLYCEMIA.

Another common myth that many people have about fasting is that it can lead to hypoglycemia. The reason this is thought is because if you aren't eating food, especially carbohydrates every few hours, your body is surely going to run into low energy levels and then if no food comes in—hypoglycemia.

Hypoglycemia is essentially what happens when blood glucose levels drop too low and not enough fuel is getting to the brain and body.

Fortunately, the body has strong protective mechanisms against this and those kick in when fasting. The reason many people get hypoglycemic in today's world is because they are constantly eating simple sugars. So, they eat a meal rich in carbs, experience the blood glucose high, and then crash shortly after that.

Then they eat more carbs, get the high again, followed by the crash. On and on this continues.

But when you fast, provided your last meal was rich in protein and healthy fats, you don't get this crash. Your body doesn't go from high blood glucose to low blood glucose. It goes from burning fatty acids from the foods you ate to burning fatty acids from your fat cells, released through the process of lipolysis (this 'fat burning' is the breakdown of stored fats and other lipids into fatty acids), and that now becomes your primary fuel source.

This is one reason why it's important on a fasting diet not to just eat all the junk food you want. Doing so could set you up for hypoglycemia if you aren't careful.

By instead focusing on some complex carbohydrates, fibrous carbohydrates, and then lots of lean protein coupled with healthy fats, you'll prime your body for fat burning.

Once you get into the state of using fat as a fuel source rather than glucose, you are no longer at risk of low blood sugar. This is also what takes place during the ketogenic diet. Some individuals who fast long enough may even move into ketosis and this is where blood glucose levels are incredibly stable.

MYTH #8: BREAKFAST IS THE MOST IMPORTANT MEAL OF THE DAY.

We've all heard this: You need to eat your breakfast! Our mothers told us when we were young and now even as adults, we may still carry that motto around.

The fact is though, breakfast is not the most important meal of the day. Your body is perfectly equipped to go without food for longer than 8 hours each day and once you train it to adapt to a new eating schedule, you'll hardly miss breakfast at all.

In fact, breakfast may be more detrimental to your health than it is good if you are looking for fat loss because you are essentially putting the brakes on fat burning. When you fast overnight, your body is going to start seeing an increase in hormone sensitive lipase, which is a hormone that directs the total amount of fat burning taking place.

What shuts this hormone off? Carbs. Even the smallest of carbs will do it, so as soon as those carbs come in, your fat burning drops dramatically. By skipping breakfast, you help ensure that this hormone stays in higher concentrations throughout the body, thus you continue to burn fat well into the morning. This can help you see far superior results than you would have if you ate breakfast.

And most people will adapt. You may find that the first day or two you do feel slightly hungry and even 'off' when you skip your morning meal. But as time progresses on, your body adapts and, soon, you'll hardly even miss breakfast.

Look at how many adults skip breakfast unintentionally just because they are so busy! Lots do, and they are just fine. So, don't be so caught up in thinking you must eat breakfast in order to see results or stay healthy. There's nothing magical about breakfast.

Research has shown that there is virtually no advantage in weight loss results when comparing breakfast eaters to those who skip breakfast2.

This said, do keep in mind that young children and teens do tend to perform better at school when they eat breakfast, so this is not the recommended strategy for anyone under the age of 18.

MYTH #9: FASTING CAUSES MALNOURISHMENT.

Another common notion is the idea that fasting will lead to malnourishment. This too is not correct. Malnourishment comes when you aren't giving the body the full spectrum of macronutrients and micronutrients it needs. That means sufficient carbohydrates, dietary fats, proteins, vitamins, and minerals.

This has nothing to do with when these nutrients come in, but more to do with whether they do—or don't—over the course of the week. You can even go a day or two without getting in the full spectrum and as long as you get more in the coming days, it'll all balance out in the end.

When you eat meals later on in the day, as long as you are getting in the same nutrient-dense foods you would have eaten earlier, just spread out, you will be sitting in the exact same position as you would with a standard meal plan. The body is still receiving those nutrients, so the only difference is when it receives them in a 24-hour period.

There is absolutely no reason at all that fasting should lead to malnourishment.

As you can see, fasting is not going to put you at any disadvantages in terms of your health and nutrition—if anything, it can actually help improve your overall standing.

The key thing to remember here is that fasting is simply a way of structuring your meal plan. It's not a prescribed diet where you have to eat this or that or eat so much of any one certain food. Choosing the right diet to implement with your fasting protocol will be key to your success. And this is exactly what we will show you with The Fasting Plan.

Chapter 3 Key Takeaways

•	Fasting will not cause you to lose muscle—in fact, the right nutrition during your fast coupled with smart exercise training can actually help you gain muscle while losing body fat.

•	Fasting can enhance many elements of your health and can help promote autophagy, thermogenesis, and support disease prevention.

•	Fasting will not deprive you of nutrients if you choose your foods wisely. Your specific food choices will have everything to do with how your body responds, nutritionally speaking, to the fast.

•	The body can continue to function just fine even if you aren't eating carbohydrates every few hours.

•	When you fast, your body is able to tap into stored fat more easily.

•	Those who don't fast and eat multiple times per day are more likely to overeat than those who do fast due to inaccurate estimations of food consumed and hunger. Fasting will actually decrease hunger in most people, making it easier to stick with your fat loss diet plan.

•	Many people will find their energy level increases when fasting thanks to the endorphins that are released. Eating is what decreases their energy level.

•	As long as you choose to consume meals rich in protein and healthy fats, especially right at the end of your eating window, there's no reason that you should suffer from blood sugar crashes during your fasting period.

•	The notion that breakfast is the most important meal of the day is not accurate. You can definitely go without eating breakfast and still be very healthy.

•	As long as you choose the same healthy foods during the fast that you would have when you weren't fasting, there's no reason to think you'll suffer from malnourishment.

REFERENCES

Chaouchi, A., Leiper, J. B., Souissi, N., Coutts, A. J., & Chamai, K. (2009, December). Effects of ramadan intermittent fasting on sports performance and training: a review. Retrieved from https://www.ncbi.nlm.nih.gov/pubmed/20029094

Dhurandhar, E. J., Dawson, J., Alcorn, A., Larsen, L. H., Thomas, E. A., Cardel, M., . . . Allison, D. B. (2014, August). The effectiveness of breakfast recommendations on weight loss: a randomized controlled trial. Retrieved from https://www.ncbi.nlm.nih.gov/pmc/articles/PMC4095657/
SUB SUBHEADING

CHAPTER 4: DIFFERENT TYPES OF FASTING

"Efficiency is doing things right; effectiveness is doing the right things."
-Peter Drucker

You've made it this far. You know what fasting is. You know why it's awesome. You've heard some myths around this amazing subject and, hopefully, we've addressed them and not only put your mind at ease, we've made you excited about the endless health advantages fasting offers you.

Now, we'll cover the different types of fasting. Because...damn. There are a lot of different ways to do this. So how the heck do you know which options are the best? How do you know what will work better than the others? Well that's why you picked up this book. Before we dive into it, the goal is to give you enough ammunition to be aware of each type of fasting and how to apply what is taught so you can get results as fast as humanly possible. My friend Kris Gethin always says, "Knowledge without mileage is bullshit." I'm bringing him up again because this train of thought has earned me much more success than I could have ever imagined. Theory without application isn't a great plan for success. Think about it: If you read thousands of books about the sport of basketball, you'd know quite a bit about it, right?

But, what if you had never actually picked up a basketball and made a visit to your local court? What if you never even shot the ball in the hoop? Think you'd be any good? Nope.

To be successful at anything, you have to combine theory and application. What looks good on paper might not work as well in the real world. I've experienced this with work, weight training, relationships, and, of course, fasting. As we cover each type of fasting technique, the pros/cons will both be included. You'll also see the documented evidence AND the real-world experience with it. With each type, you'll find the following three variables with a rating scale of 1 to 10. 10 being the highest/best rating and 1 being the lowest/worst rating.

EFFECTIVENESS:

How effective is it? Does it work? How well?

ADHERENCE:

How easy is it to stick with it? This is such an under-rated variable to consider when engaging in any diet or fitness program for that matter. If something works, great. But, if you hate it, are you going to stick with it long term? For me, the goal of any successful program has to have a high adherence score. It doesn't have to be easy, but it does have to be something you won't give up on. No matter how great a program is, it won't work unless you keep using the thing.

HEALTHINESS:

Health Risks? Is it healthy? Are there any side effects? Any health risks?

Finally, you'll find a quick note from me regarding my real-world experience with it. I won't be sugar coating anything and I'll give you my unbiased opinion. Keep in mind, my primary goal is to improve my health and my secondary goals are vanity. I've been in the search of a dieting lifestyle that allows simple and reproducible results for living a long, healthy life. And, if I can look good too, that's icing on the cake. Feel good and look good? Yeah. I'll take it.

Sometimes I'm longwinded, but I don't care. I'd rather nail these points home with a sledgehammer, so you know this stuff inside and out. The better I'm able to teach you, the more successful you're going to be. This won't be a diet. It'll be a way of life that will STAY with you for life. With this all being said, let's journey on and check these different types of fasting out.

WATER FASTING:

What it is:

Water fasting is voluntarily abstaining from food while consuming nothing else except for water. No supplements. No vegetables. No creamer in your coffee. Just water. Some exceptions might be the consumption of tea (depending on who's opinion you're asking).

Water fasting has been around since the beginning of time. It's the most common definition of fasting. When anyone mentions a fast, they are usually defaulting to 'water fasting'.

You might try this if you're fasting for religious reasons. Or, your doctor might have you do this if you're preparing for surgery. It's great for detoxification and has great health benefits. There are several studies that have linked water fasting with impressive health benefits (Alirezaei et al. 2010) (Castello et al. 2010) (Brandhorst et al. 2015).

How do you do it?

Water fasts don't last longer than 24-72 hours, on average, and it's recommended that you don't engage in a water fast any longer than this without proper medical guidance.

Three-days before trying water fasting, increase your water intake. Try to aim for at least 1-gallon. A good way to see if you're properly hydrated is to check the color of your urine. If it's clear, there's a higher probability you're not dehydrated.

When you decide to break your fast, most recommendations are to start with a smaller meal of nutrient-dense foods and/or a smoothie of some sort. You can start introducing bigger meals in the day as you get more comfortable.

The longer you fast, the more careful you want to be when you decide on the meal you break your fast with. There have been reported instances of re-feeding syndrome, a condition where your body undergoes rapid changes in fluid and electrolytes (Mehanna, Melodina, & Travis, 2008). From what I've seen and read, this is for extreme cases of malnourished folks undergoing prolonged periods of fasting. This is another reason why we recommend having a physician monitor you if you decide to fast longer than 72-hours. While it's not common, it's important you're aware.

Other popular names for water fasting are: "The Lemon Detox Cleanse". You only consume a mixture of lemon juice, water, maple syrup, and cayenne pepper, several times per day for up to 7-days (Shetty, Mooventhan, & Nagendra, 2016). However, it is my opinion that including any calories in your period of time restricted eating window means you aren't water fasting.

Effectiveness: 10/10

Water fasting has been shown to promote autophagy, so your body can engage in cell regeneration. It has also been shown to promote fat-loss, improved insulin sensitivity for hypertrophy (muscle-gain) and many other awesome things.

Adherence: 3/10

This is the rub. Do you want to not eat for extended periods of time? Think you can sustain not eating for 72-hours often? Does it sound fun? Nope. Not to me. While there are a few people out there who can actually stick to water fasting, most find it too difficult/boring to adhere to. Another thing—fast this long and you might notice you're pretty irritable. And if I'm unable to have my coffee and creamer, it makes it pretty damn difficult to stick to the program. Just remember everyone is different so I recommend trying these methods out yourself if you're curious. However, I believe I've found a better way to fast, which is why you're reading this book.

Healthiness: 10/10

This gets a very high score for the health side too. You really can't beat water fasting. It gives your body's digestive system a break, so it can focus on autophagy (cell-cleansing), thermogenesis, and disease prevention while promoting improved insulin sensitivity.

Overall Score: 23/30

Water fasting kicks ass. However, the adherence score is very low. It doesn't matter how good a program is if you can't/don't stick to it. I've competed in various bodybuilding shows and the diets are difficult. They worked too, but do you think I wanted to eat boring food that had little to zero taste all my life? Nope. I like to work hard and play hard.

The goal is to enjoy life and all it has to offer. I don't want to eat out of Tupperware and I don't want to only be able to drink water while I watch all my friends and family have tasty, delicious food at Thanksgiving. If your friends ask you to have a beer with them, don't you want to be able to have the freedom to do what you want? Look, it doesn't matter if drink or don't drink. The point is to provide you with an option that gives you total control over your life. With this autonomy, the odds of you finding more happiness are much higher.

DRY FASTING:

What it is:

Dry fasting entails abstaining from the consumption of food and water for a limited period of time. It's not as popular as water fasting and the idea alone scares people from trying it.

It is popular with some religions, especially Muslims during the month of Ramadan. Animals have also been known to instinctively use dry fasting to heal themselves. When hurt or sick, they seek shelter away from outside influences and purposely avoid water and food until they feel better.

There are generally a few different names for dry fasting.

1.	Soft Dry Fast: In this fast, folks can have 'soft' contact with water. This means they can take showers and brush their teeth with water, but they still abstain from drinking.

2.	Absolute Dry Fast: In this approach, you aren't allowed to have any contact with water whatsoever. No Showers. No baths. No consumption.

It's also worth noting there are two forms of dry fasting. "Intermittent dry fasting" generally means water consumption is only allowed for small periods and the remainder of the day is reserved for complete fasting. The other form of dry fasting is "prolonged dry fasting". This is where folks will voluntarily avoid food for periods longer than 24-hours.

How do you do it?

During the day, some will avoid consuming any food or water during the daylight (usually 12-hours). It was popularized by religious cultures to teach those who practice dry fasting more discipline and control in their lives and bring them closer to God. Other religions who practice dry fasting are: Christians, Jews, and Mormons, to name a few.

One way of practicing dry fasting is as follows: Consume a normal meal at breakfast then avoid food and water for the remainder of the day. They will usually dry fast for approximately 8-10 hours and resume eating and drinking later in the evening. Alternatively, it is said you can safely use "prolonged dry fasting" for 24-36 hours and reap the benefits.

[*NOTE: I do not claim to be a doctor. Please consult your doctor before trying any technique or recommendation found in this book.*]

Effectiveness: 10/10

Dry fasting has amazing benefits and is very similar to water fasting. On top of the added benefits of neuroprotection (an effect that may result in salvaging, recovering, or regeneration of the nervous system's cells, structure, and function), cell-regeneration, and disease prevention, it is said that dry fasting can even further enhance the cleansing process without dehydrating you. If you do it right, you may help your body to burn more fat.

It never ceases to amaze us of what the human body is capable of. By eliminating water and food intake, the body undergoes a certain amount of stress and is forced to create its own nutrients and water and metabolizes fat. Just about every organ of your body goes into 'work-mode' and contributes to the process of cell repair and regeneration.

Adherence: 2/10

While dry fasting is extremely effective, it's almost impossible to maintain for extended periods of time (and not recommended for extended periods of time either). Irritability is even higher than water fasting. Think about it: You can't consume anything at all. That sucks. I'd be pissed off too if I had to watch my friends drink a damn glass of water while I had to watch paint dry. However, if you are able to combine this with other forms of fasting with higher adherence scores, your chances of success will be much higher!

Healthiness: 10/10

If you do this right, you will experience the same results as water fasting with the added benefit of an even more enhanced process of cell-cleansing, thermogenesis, and autophagy. And that's only naming a few benefits—the list goes on.

Overall Score: 22/30

While this score is only one point less than the overall score of water fasting, this form of fasting is extremely effective, and it has its place in any solid fasting program, in my honest opinion. It's hard as hell to adhere to though. No one wants to go without food or water. However, if you're able to properly incorporate dry fasting into your routine, your results will follow. It can also be dangerous for you.

INTERMITTENT FASTING

What it is:

in·ter·mit·tent
adjective: intermittent
1.   occurring at irregular intervals; not continuous or
steady.

As the word 'intermittent' implies, intermittent fasting
involves periods of time-restricted eating at irregular
intervals. This can lead to some confusion as to what people
truly mean when they throw the term "intermittent fasting"
around with their peers because people make it more
complicated than it really is.

The time-restricted eating periods can vary a great deal
between which form of intermittent fasting you decide to
take part in. Below, we will discuss the more popular forms
of intermittent fasting. Note that you can combine
intermittent fasting with dry fasting and/or water fasting.

How do you do it?

There are many variations of intermittent fasting. We will
cover some of the most popular variations and provide
ratings for each. Since there are many variations, we will
focus on the most popular forms regarding the ratings of
effectiveness, adherence and effectiveness.

THE 16/8 VARIATION

What it is:

- In this variation, you fast for 16-hours and your feeding
window is limited to an 8-hour period. There isn't a specific
time you have to begin fasting. What matters is that you

ensure you fast for 16-hours and your feeding window is under the 8-hour period of time.

How do you do it?

How you do it really depends on your schedule and what works best for you. It doesn't matter which hours of the day you decide to fast. It only matters that you maintain a 16-hour period of time-restricted eating. Try skipping breakfast. If you work out, try doing it in the early morning after waking. Try scheduling your feeding window between 2 pm and 10 pm. During this 8-hour period, you can eat as many meals as you like. What you eat isn't as important as when you eat it.

Effectiveness 9/10

If you are going to fast, it is recommended that you at least provide yourself with a solid 16-hour window of time. Every time you eat, you spike your insulin levels. If you're able to at least go 16 hours without eating, you're able to take advantage of your body's thermogenesis (fat burning) capabilities. The 16/8 method is fantastic. I give it a 9/10 rating.

Adherence 10/10

This is insanely easy to stick to. Think about it. If you stop eating at 8 pm, you wouldn't eat again until 12 pm the next day. All you need to do is skip breakfast the next day. If you use the methods in this program, you'll start understanding true hunger and this will be a breeze. More on this in the chapters to come.

Healthiness 10/10

The 16/8 method of fasting continues to earn it's place in the fasting community and is quickly becoming one of the best way's to fast. In one study, folks who employed the 16/8 method consumed 350 fewer calories, lost 3 percent of their weight, and had lower blood pressure.

Overall score: 29/30.

The 16/8 method kicks ass and for that reason, you will be using a variation of it when you use this program.

THE EAT-STOP-EAT VARIATION

What it is:

This form of fasting allows a 24-hour fast. Like the 16/8 variation, the specific time of day you decide to fast isn't important. All that matters is that you fast for 24-hours total. It's also called 'eat-stop-eat' fasting because you eat your last meal, then fast for 24-hours, and finally break your fast with another meal. In this variation, you fast 1-2 times per week.

How do you do it?

The most popular way to use the 'eat-stop-eat' fast is as follows: After you finish your dinner in the evening, you'll begin the full 24-hour fast until dinner time the following day where you break your fast. Alternatively, you can employ the same strategy by beginning the 24-hour fast after breakfast and not eating again until the same time the next day. It is common for folks to use the 'eat-stop-eat' fast twice per week.

Effectiveness 6/10

Don't let the rating fool you. This is a very effective form of fasting. I've seen folks get good results with this form of fasting. However, fasting only 1-2 times per week doesn't provide your body with the same amount of time in a fasted state. And remember, this is where the magic happens.

Adherence 7/10

Most people don't like fasting for 24 hours. If you don't do something regularly, it's much more difficult and less enjoyable to do. In my experience, I end up dreading the 24 hours leading up to the fast because it's only 1-2 times per week. I like to think of this in the way of creating a workout routine. If you only go to the gym once a week, it makes it very hard to develop a solid habit. On the contrary, if you try working out 3-4 times per week, you'll notice yourself easing into a very valuable routine and it becomes an enjoyable part of your lifestyle.

Healthiness 10/10

Fasting for 24 hours has proven to be quite healthy.

Overall score: 23/30

This is a great variation of fasting and can prove to be quite effective for a good amount of people. However, it is much more difficult to develop a structured routine.

THE 5/2 VARIATION

What it is:

During this diet, you intermittently fast twice per week and eat normally on the other days. On the fasting days, your calories are reduced to ~600 for men and ~500 for women.

How do you do it?

The rules are as follows: You only have to fast twice per week and can pick any days you like. Just ensure the fasting days aren't planned consecutively. During the fasting days, you can eat whenever you want but you can't eat more than 500-600 calories. A popular way to do this is to fast on Monday and Thursday and eat normally during the other days of the week.

During your fasting days, folks have found it easier to fast for most of the day and finally eat the majority of your calories in one meal. Doing this will give you a greater sense of fullness and your satiety hormone in your brain will have a greater chance of kicking in. If you were to break up the calories into 3-4 smaller meals, it may be more difficult for you to get through these days.

Effectiveness 6/10

I rated this 6/10 because it's so hard to adhere to. No program, no matter how effective it is, will be successful if you're aren't able to stick to it.

Adherence 5/10

In my opinion, this is harder to stick to compared to other forms of fasting. During the 'fasted' days, you're required to eat 600 calories. Eating this much might just make you hungrier. If you want to be lean long term, you want to find a way of eating that doesn't leave you with a feeling of deprivation.

Healthiness 9/10

Fasting 24 hours is great. Eating whatever you want during the week might not be (depending on what you're choosing to eat).

Overall score: 20/30

In controlled fasting, I recommend eating little to no calories during your fast. I suggest to keep calories at 200 or less. This allows you to eat enough food to help with hunger/satiety while keeping your insulin low enough to allow your body to do it's magic. And when I say eating enough food to help you terminate hunger, the type of food is important too. I feel that eating 600 calories might negate the effects of what you're trying to accomplish. I also feel it just teases my hunger and makes it harder to adhere to. This wouldn't work well for me over long periods of time. However, if this works well for you, go for it. After all, we are all different. Everyone needs to experiment and use what works best for them.

THE 4/3 VARIATION (ALTERNATE DAY FASTING)

What it is:

Also known as 'alternate day fasting', in the 4/3 diet you fast one day, resume eating normal meals the following day, and follow the same alternating schedule for the entire week. It's similar to the 5/2 diet in that you eat a maximum of 500-600 calories on your fasting days.

How do you do it?

Begin eating normal meals on Monday. Once you've finished dinner, the 24-hour fast begins and ends on the same time the following day. It's recommended that you try fasting for most of the day and save the majority of the 500-600 calories for one bigger meal to make it easier to survive these more difficult days.

Effectiveness 7/10

I'm giving this one with an 7/10 for effectiveness based on my own experience with it. I've found that it works almost as well as the 16/8. Depending on how you look at it, this method allows you to fast 3-4 days per week while the 16/8 method requires you to fast everyday if you wish to do so. It is my preference to give your body a larger fasting period of time as often as possible. See table 3.1. In this example, we are assuming you fast Tuesday, Thursday and Saturday with the 'eat, stop eat' variation. In this case, you'd give your body a total of 72 hours to work it's magic. Alternatively, the 16/8 will provide you with a larger amount of time in a fasted state (112 hours). It also forces you to incorporate fasting into your daily routine. In my opinion, this helps solidify your understanding of true hunger compared to emotional hunger. This is very powerful, especially if your goal is to stay lean indefinitely

	Mon	Tue	Wed	Thur	Fri	Sat	Sun	Total Fasting Hours
Eat/Stop/Eat	NO FAST	24	NO FAST	24	NO FAST	24	NO FAST	72 hours
16/8	16	16	16	16	16	16	16	112 hours

Figure 3.1

Adherence 8/10.

Most people who try this either love or hate this variation. There is no grey area. For some, it is very difficult to fast for 24 hours. Others find it to be easy.

Healthiness 10/1

No surprise here. It's very healthy to give your body time to detoxify and dedicate its resources to thermogenesis.

Overall rating: 25/30

This is a great option for a lot of people. It's easy to work in their schedules. However, it is my opinion that it isn't as great as the 16/8 due to the reasons explained above.

CHAPTER 3 KEY TAKEAWAYS

There are many forms of fasting and to be completely candid, they are all effective in their own way. When you decide on which method is best for you, try using the rating system for yourself by testing effectiveness, adherence and healthiness. I'd never be brash and tell you that there is only one way to do something. Since everyone is different, I suggest that you do what you think works best for you. However, the reason I believe the fasting plan to be the most optimal solution is due to the amazing benefits and the amount of work you're required to put into it. In other words, it provides you with the best bang for the buck.

CHAPTER REFERENCES

Trepanowski JF1, Kroeger CM2 (2017, July). Effect of Alternate-Day Fasting on Weight Loss, Weight Maintenance, and Cardioprotection Among Metabolically Healthy Obese Adults: A Randomized Clinical Trial. Retrieved from https://www.ncbi.nlm.nih.gov/pubmed/28459931

Alirezaei, M., Kemball, C. C., Flynn, C. T., Wood, M. R., Whitton, J. L., & Kiosses, W. B. (2010, August). Short-term fasting induces profound neuronal autophagy. Retrieved from https://www.ncbi.nlm.nih.gov/pmc/articles/PMC3106288/

Castello, L., Froio, T., Maina, M., Cavallini, G., Biasi, F., Leonarduzzi, G., . . . Chiarpotto, E. (2010, January). Alternate-day fasting protects the rat heart against age-induced inflammation and fibrosis by inhibiting oxidative damage and NF-kB activation. Retrieved from https://www.ncbi.nlm.nih.gov/pubmed/19818847/

Brandhorst, S., Choi, I. Y., Wei, M., Cheng, C. W., Sedrakryan, S., Navarrete, G., . . . Longo, V. D. (2015, July). A periodic diet that mimics fasting promotes multi-system regeneration, enhanced cognitive performance and healthspan. Retrieved from https://www.ncbi.nlm.nih.gov/pmc/articles/PMC4509734/

Mehanna, H. M., Moledina, J., & Travis, J. (2008, June).
Refeeding syndrome: what it is, and how to prevent and treat
it. Retrieved from
https://www.ncbi.nlm.nih.gov/pmc/articles/PMC2440847/

Shetty, P., Mooventhan, A., & Nagendra, H. R. (2016, March).
Does short-term lemon honey juice fasting have effect on
lipid profile and body composition in healthy individuals?.
Retrieved from
https://www.ncbi.nlm.nih.gov/pmc/articles/PMC4910284/

PART II: HOW TO START FASTING

"Success is neither magical or mysterious. Success is the
natural consequence of consistently applying the basic
fundamentals."
-Jim Rohn

There is no magic program that will cease to defy the laws of
physiology. Meaning, there is no one magic pill or program
that will make you instantly achieve your goals. However,
there are systems that have been developed over time that
have been shown to work better than others to help you
achieve your goals faster. Then, there are the unicorns out
there that reap huge rewards for the least amount of work.
This is where The Fasting Plan comes in. I've never found a
better system to get you in shape fast as hell while living a
normal life (as much of a normal life I can imagine lol). Yep—
this program kicks major ass. But remember: It only works if
you do.

Before you begin this program, you need to understand the
basics. Once you learn the basics, work hard to master them
by applying what you learn every single day.

The difference between successful and unsuccessful people is
the simple idea of execution. If you're able to execute the
principles being taught here optimally, you will get results
much faster. Many forget the idea of execution and these
folks might get short-term results but never change their

lives. And they never reach the potential they hoped for. Don't be one of these fools. Life is too short so master this shit and turn some heads. Let's get to it.

I've separated the following topics into their respective chapters for your convenience. When you use this program, you'll be able to go right back to each section when and if you need to. Think of this as a study guide and use these suggestions as much as possible.

WHAT TO KNOW ABOUT EATING (WHEN YOU'RE NOT FASTING)

Chapter : 5 The Basics of Nutrition

What a Healthy Diet Is
How your body burns fat
Calories, Macro-, and Micro-nutrients Defined
How to Count Macronutrients

WHAT TO KNOW ABOUT FASTING

Chapter 6: Controlled fasting

What Breaks a Fast
Fasting and Hunger: how to deal with it.
What to Include During Fasting
What to Avoid During Fasting

HOW TO START FASTING

Chapter 5. The Basics Of Nutrition

> "Our food should be our medicine and our medicine should
> be our food. "
> -Hippocrates

What a Healthy Diet Is

I'm probably telling you something you already know: Eating healthy is better than eating unhealthy. Duh. But what does this really mean? We all know veggies are good and fat is bad, right? No. Fats aren't bad. In my opinion, healthy food is food that is high in nutrient density, meaning fiber, phytonutrients, and micronutrients. Unhealthy food is food that is processed. Food you'll find in the grocery store that is boxed usually includes ingredients designed to enhance the shelf life of the product. These ingredients usually aren't healthy. Boxed food is dead food. From this point on, think of healthy food as food that is alive and unhealthy food is dead food.

The Importance of Nutrient-Dense Food

This idea isn't rocket science, but most people will disregard it. Even if you know nothing of dieting or nutrition, I'm willing to bet you know what NOT to eat. If you want to get in better shape, you know enough not to eat fast food in every meal. You know vegetables are good for you and contain vitamins, right? My point is to trust yourself a little bit more.

Use your judgement and critical thinking skills when you select the food you supply your body with.

When we talk about nutrient-dense foods, we are talking about foods that nourish your body, health, and mind. They give you the most bang for the buck. The benefits they provide are far superior to the caloric return you get back from eating them. Nutrient-dense foods also make you feel much fuller than foods that contain empty calories. This means you can eat more nutrient-dense foods and feel much fuller and more satisfied after eating them. I call these nutrient-dense options: High Volume Foods.

If you are a Formula One racecar driver, you want to fuel your racecar with the highest-octane fuel you can find. You know that it will make your car run better and ultimately help make the difference between winning and losing races. Your body is the same way. Pick foods that are highly nutritious and packed with vitamins, minerals, and fiber. Your digestion system will thank you for it. Your energy levels will pay you rewards, and your mental capacity and long-term health will benefit you.

The following are some suggestions for nutrient-dense foods. Try including them in your diet, especially when fasting. But, so I'm clear, nutrient-dense foods will benefit you no matter what type of diet you are engaged in. The following foods are only suggestions.

VEGGIES:

Kale
Spinach
Kale
Seaweed
Garlic
Parsley
Asparagus
Bok Choy
Brussel Sprouts
Tomatoes
Carrots

CARBS:

Potatoes
Blueberries
Strawberries
Raspberries
Honey
Acai Berries
Elder Berries
Goji Berries

PROTEIN:

Salmon
Shellfish
Liver
Sardines
Eggs
Whey Protein Isolate
Collagen Protein

FATS:

Coconut oil
MCT Oil
Lecithin
Omega 3 and 6 fats
Chia Seeds
Flax seeds
Fermented Drinks:
Kombucha

You'll need to experiment with which foods you like better and stick with the foods you enjoy the most. For example, I enjoy salads made of kale, spinach, peppers, carrots, and salmon. I'll sprinkle in blueberries, raspberries strawberries, etc. depending on the day. Mix and match however fits you the best. Have fun with this!

How Your Body Burns Fat

If you understand the idea of weight loss/fat burning, you'll be in a much more advantageous position and you're going to have a higher chance of making this fasting stuff work well for you.

No matter what diet you are using, you need to understand: In order to lose fat, you need to eat less calories than your body uses. The opposite is true for building muscle. If you want to gain weight, you have to eat more calories than your body uses. Today, I'm keeping this idea general, but I want you to understand the way I think. This is very simple, yet many people miss the importance of this idea and still don't understand why they can't get that six-pack, no matter how hard they try.

Think about it. No diet, no matter how awesome it is, will give you results unless you pay attention to this fact. I'm going to repeat it because your success depends on it!

EAT LESS than you burn = Fat/weight loss.

EAT MORE than you burn = Muscle/weight gain.

Think about this analogy. There's a plane flying through the sky. The plane is burning fuel while it's moving. If we added gas to this plane, we'd stop once the fuel tank was full, or else the gas would spill out (i.e. go to waste and not get used). We'd only add gas to the plane again until the tank started running out of gas. If we were going give the plane extra fuel, we would add extra fuel to the reserve tanks on the plane. Once the reserve tanks were full, there's no tanks to fill. Any extra gas we give the plane is wasted.

Think of your body the same way. Our body is always burning calories. Once we've filled it with macronutrients, we have a full tank and don't need anymore. If we eat MORE food than our body requires, the extra calories will go to waste (and possibly fat gain). If we want to build muscle, we need to eat more food (fill our reserve tanks just like the plane). But once our reserve tanks are full, any extra food is not going to benefit us—it will be wasted (and we'll gain unwanted weight/fat).

To illustrate this even further, let's take a 180lb man. Let's say his maintenance calories are 2,000 per day. This means he needs to eat 2,000 calories to stay the same weight.

If he wants to lose fat/lose weight, he'll need to eat less. For example, he'd eat 1,900 calories. The loss of 100 calories creates a calorie deficit and helps him burn fat.

If he wants to gain muscle, he'd eat more calories. For example, he'd eat 2,100 calories. These extra 100 calories go to his reserve tank (creates a calorie surplus) and helps him build muscle.

There's a lot more to it than this, but the basic idea of how calories (macronutrients) work will help you get closer to your goals. If you want to manipulate your calories to burn fat, you now understand the foundation. If you want to use macronutrients to build muscle, you know how to do that too.

These are starting points. The way you're going to improve has to do with tracking changes your body makes over time. I can give you theories and more complicated strategies. However, I feel giving you a starting point will serve you better because it will teach you how to make changes depending on what your body does over time instead of making changes based off what someone else told you to do. Your body is smarter than we are, so work with it, not against it.

Note: Once you get to the Fat Burning Fasting Plan, you won't be tracking calories or macros. This section is put together to get you to understand how your body burns fat. The Fat Burning Fasting Plan will teach you how to eat in a way that is easier to stick to. More on that later...

CALORIES, MACRO-, AND MICRO-NUTRIENTS DEFINED

Calories are the units of energy you get from food. Macronutrients are the calories you are consuming. They are as follows: Protein, Carbohydrates, and Fats. Anytime you eat food, calories come from one of these three macronutrients.

1 gram of protein = 4 calories

1 gram of carbohydrate = 4 calories

1 gram of fat = 9 calories

Proteins are the building blocks of muscle and life in general. Without protein, our body wouldn't be able to build and repair itself. Every cell in the human body contains protein. This being said, we need to eat protein to sustain this process. So, protein isn't just important for meatheads and bodybuilders—it's important for everyone. For every gram of protein, we get four calories.

Foods that contain protein are poultry, meat, seafood, fish, eggs, and legumes. There are many more sources of protein but, for our purposes, just think of protein as meat. If you're vegan, think of protein as tofu, peas, or soy.

Carbohydrates provide you with energy and fuel for your daily activities and workouts. Each gram of carbohydrate provides 4 calories per gram consumed; good examples of carbohydrates are bread, pasta, veggies, rice, lentils, and sweet potatoes.

Dietary fat is also a great fuel source for daily activity. Each gram of fat provides 9 calories. Dietary fat is different than fat stored in the body. Just about every piece of food you can think of contains fat. Keep in mind that the calories per gram is more than double the calories of other macronutrients so it's much easier to get more fat in your diet. There are different types of fat. For the sake of brevity, we will discuss the basics of saturated and unsaturated fats.

Saturated Fats: These are fats found mostly in animal products and packaged products. Examples of saturated fats are those found in steak, seafood, eggs, and other fatty-cuts of meats. In this program, it's perfectly acceptable to eat fat from animal products. The fat that you'll want to avoid, if possible, is packaged foods like potato chips, ice cream, and other fatty snack foods.

When in doubt, buy foods at your local grocery store by shopping around the perimeter of the store. For the most part, stay away from the foods located in the other parts of the store. Canned food of any kind is usually not the best option. However, it's not the end of the world if you do eat it every once in a while. Just try to eat whole foods when you can. The reason is simple: Whole foods that are found in the perimeter of the grocery store are generally the most nutrient dense. Think of these foods in the same way you'd think of high-octane racecar fuel compared to the lowest-grade fuel. Your automobile will function on low-grade fuel, but it isn't optimal. If you want to keep your body and car in the best shape, fuel it with the best grade of fuel!

MAINTENANCE CALORIES

Before calculating your macronutrients, you need to know the amount of maintenance calories required for your body to sustain day to day activities. Once you figure this number out, you'll be in a more advantageous position to lose fat.

Your maintenance calories are what you need to stay exactly the same weight. There are many different types of equations that will give you estimates of what this should be. Instead of giving you an equation, I prefer to recommend taking action by eating normally for 3-5 days. This means that you'll try and eat the same types of foods you normally do at the same normal times. Keep track of the foods you eat and record the quantities consumed. You can either write them down or use an app to track your macros. I prefer 'My Fitness Pal." It's free and it's very easy to use. The idea is to get an understanding of what you are eating and take the average over 3 days or 5 days. In my opinion, this will give you the most accurate idea of your maintenance calorie level.

For example, let's say you are a man and have tracked your calorie consumption for 3 days. You get the following:

Day 1: 2,341 calories

Day 2: 2,456 calories

Day 3: 2, 654 calories

Take the average of the three days by diving the total by the number of calories consumed by the total number of days. Ex. (2,341 + 2,456, + 2654 = 7,451. 7,451 divided by 3 days = 2,483.6 calories per day).

Now that you have a basic understanding of finding your maintenance calories, you can calculate your macros.

HOW TO COUNT MACRONUTRIENTS:

STEP ONE: CALCULATING PROTEIN

Recent studies have shown you need between 1.3 to 1.8 grams of protein per kilogram of body weight (.6 to .8 grams of protein per pound of body weight) to maximize muscle protein synthesis and build muscle. If you're an athlete, higher protein may be warranted depending on other variables like training intensity, training frequency, carbohydrate availability, and training history (Phillips & Van Loon, 2011) (Lemon, 2000) (Helms, Zinn, Rowlands, & Brown, 2013).

Now you know the numbers. To make things easy, I've always preferred to err on the side of caution and keep protein at 1 to 1.2 grams per pound of bodyweight. When cutting (burning fat) I've found that keeping protein high makes me less hungry. When building muscle, I've found that keeping protein at this same level maximizes my chances for success. For these reasons, the amount of protein I suggest is 1 gram of protein per pound of bodyweight.

Question: Since the studies say to keep protein between .6 and .8 grams of protein per bodyweight, can I reduce my protein to this?

Answer: Absolutely. The reason I like keeping protein at 1 gram per pound is simplicity. I feel it doesn't hurt anything by staying at this number. It also keeps my satiety up, especially when dieting (and calories are in a deficit). I hate being hungry and higher protein helps me stay fuller for longer. If you find eating less protein works better for you, go ahead and lower it. Do what works for you.

Recall earlier:

1 gram of protein = 4 calories

Weigh yourself and get your bodyweight. This is equal to your required grams of protein needed each day. Example: if you weight 200 pounds, you'd need to consume 200 grams of protein.

Since you need 1 gram per pound of bodyweight, we need to multiply 200 grams by 4 (1 gram protein = 4 calories) to equal 800 calories. Next, subtract this number from your total calories (In our example, 2,000 - 800 = 1,200 calories).

To reiterate:

1. Total bodyweight = grams of protein. (i.e. 200lb man = 200 grams protein)

2. Total protein x 4 = total calories coming from protein (200 x 4 = 800)

3. Total calories - total protein calories (2,000 - 800 = 1,200)

The total protein needed for each day is 200 grams or 800 calories.

STEP TWO: CALCULATING FATS

It is recommended that the daily intake of fat be between 20% and 35% for healthy adults (See below if you're interested in viewing the references.)

Office of Disease Prevention and Health Promotion. Dietary Guidelines for Americans 2010 Accessed 12/3/2014.

I've always felt very comfortable keeping my fat intake around 30 percent of my daily calories. This is a good starting point for most people for general health and satiety.

Recall earlier that:

1 gram of fat = 9 calories per gram

Multiply your total calories by .3 (30 percent).

In our example, our total calories are equal to 2,000 (2,000 x .3 = 600). To get your total grams of fat, divide the total fat calories by 9 (600 / 9 = 66.66). Then round that number to the nearest whole (66.66 = 67 grams of fat.)

Subtract the total fat calories from your total. (In our example, we'd subtract 600 from 1,200, for 600 daily calories left).

To reiterate:

Total grams of fat x .3 = 30 percent of calories coming from fat (2,000 x .3 = 600)

Total calories of fat / 9 = total grams of fat (600 / 9 = approximately 67 grams of fat)

Total calories - total calories of fat (1,200 - 600 = 600).

Above, we started with 2,000 calories. We figured out our total protein and subtracted it from our total, giving us 1,200 calories. Then, we calculated our total fat calories (600) and subtracted that from our total, giving us 600 calories left.

STEP THREE: CALCULATING CARBOHYDRATES

Recall earlier that:

1 gram carbohydrate = 4 calories

We already figured out our protein and fat calories. We are left with 600 calories (~67 grams of fat).

600 calories / 4 = 150 carbs

In our example, we are left with the current macros:

Protein = 200 grams

Fat = 67 grams

Carbohydrate = 150 grams

Now you know how to calculate your total macros for the day.

Recall that in order to burn fat, you need to be in a calorie deficit. Since everyone is different, it is tough to tell you what number you need to reduce calories by. However, it is important that you know you'll need to eat less calories than your body burns in order to lose fat.

CHAPTER SUMMARY

Nutrient dense food is healthy food. If you want to get in shape and stay in shape, you'll want to choose this as your first option.

Boxed food is dead food. From this point on, think of healthy food as food that is alive and unhealthy food is dead food. When shopping for food, try and choose foods located in the perimeters of the grocery store and try to avoid processed foods.

Your body burns fat if you're eating less calories than it's using. This means you need to be in a calorie deficit. No diet will work to help you burn fat unless you understand this important point.

EAT LESS than you burn = Fat/weight loss.

EAT MORE than you burn = Muscle/weight gain.

Maintenance calories are the calories your body requires to sustain day to day activities. There are many ways to find your maintenance calories. I prefer keeping track of what you eat for a few days and simply obtaining an average.

Macronutrients are how you get calories. Understand that:
1 gram of protein = 4 calories
1 gram of carbohydrate = 4 calories
1 gram of fat = 9 calories

How to count macronutrients. Begin by figuring out your total protein requirements. You can start by using 1 gram of protein per pound of bodyweight. Next, you'll need to calculate your fats. You can do this by multiplying your total calories by .30.

CHAPTER REFERENCES

Phillips, S. M., & Van Loon, L. J. (2011). Dietary protein for athletes: from requirements to optimum adaptation. Retrieved from https://www.ncbi.nlm.nih.gov/pubmed/22150425

Lemon, P. W. (2000, October). Beyond the zone: protein needs of active individuals. Retrieved from https://www.ncbi.nlm.nih.gov/pubmed/11023001

Helms, E. R., Zinn, C., Rowlands, D. S., & Brown, S. R. (2013, October). A systematic review of dietary protein during caloric restriction in resistance trained lean athletes: a case for higher intakes. Retrieved from https://www.researchgate.net/publication/257350851_A_S ystematic_Review_of_Dietary_Protein_During_Caloric_Restric tion_in_Resistance_Trained_Lean_Athletes_A_Case_for_Higher _Intakes

Kinsey, A. W., & Ormsbee, M. J. (2015, April). The health impact of nighttime eating: old and new perspectives. Retrieved from https://www.ncbi.nlm.nih.gov/pmc/articles/PMC4425165/

Reid, K. J., Baron, K. G., & Zee, P. C. (2014, November). Meal timing influences daily caloric intake in healthy adults.

Retrieved from
https://www.ncbi.nlm.nih.gov/pubmed/25439026

Spaeth, A. M., Dinges, D. F., & Goel, N. (2013, July). Effects of
experimental sleep restriction on weight gain, caloric intake,
and meal timing in healthy adults. Retrieved from
https://www.ncbi.nlm.nih.gov/pubmed/23814334

CHAPTER 6. CONTROLLED FASTING

"We never repent of having eaten too little."
-Thomas Jefferson

Controlled fasting, as originally described by Ori Hofmekler in his popular book 'The Warrior Diet', is based on eating under one-full meal during the under-eating phase of fasting. In the Fasting Plan, we will take it one step further and define controlled fasting as eating 'little to no food' during the under-eating phase. You are allowed to eat a maximum of 200 calories during this phase. While you are allowed to consume calories, with controlled fasting, you are allowed to have some calories during the day if you are absolutely starving and need to curb your hunger in order to make it to the finish line. I want you to do everything you can to abstain from food during the fasting period. More on how to apply controlled fasting in the chapters to come.

By practicing this form of controlled fasting, you will be disciplining yourself by strengthening your resolve. The goal is to teach you to understand your body and learn what true hunger is and what it is not. Throughout the years, we've been conditioned to eat 3-6 meals per day because our culture has taught us this is the norm. There are many people out there who just aren't hungry in the morning and try to force feed themselves because they've been taught that: 'Breakfast is the most important meal of the day.' There are also people out there who just aren't hungry when dinner-time rolls around and still think they need to eat a massive dinner. Then, there are those out there who are hungry all the time and all they think about is food. With the fasting program, your whole body will get better and better with the identification of hunger and start auto-regulating itself to instinctively know if you're really hungry or not. And this is where the magic happens. If you know what true hunger is, of course your body will start functioning more optimally.

You know that eating more calories than your body burns will help you add additional pounds to your frame. Instead of creating a surplus of unused calories all the time, you'll start eating only the calories you need because of how well you understand your body. Think of your body as a car: If you fill the gas tank of your car 3-times a day (i.e. breakfast, lunch, and dinner) but you aren't driving the car anywhere, would any of this make sense? Would the gas be put to use or would it just be wasted? If you are driving the car all over the place, obviously, you know exactly when to add more gas because the gas tank meter will show you. The more you start using controlled fasting, your internal gas tank will tell you exactly when to add more fuel. You'll only use what you need, and you'll become more efficient.

With this type of controlled fasting, I've seen success rates skyrocket because it also allows more adherence, meaning it has made it easier for folks to stick to the program. Candidly, fasting is not easy, and I never said it would be. It works but it's also quite difficult to stick to. The goal of The Fasting Plan is to create a simple and reproducible program folks can incorporate into their life easily and stick to it forever.

Controlled fasting can help you auto-regulate your hunger and optimize your calories consumed, making you an optimal machine. It will also make your life easier because it will now be something you'll be able to adhere to.

WHAT BREAKS A FAST? FOR REAL…

When you consume anything that isn't water, metabolic enzymes are created in your liver and gut. These enzymes are on a clock. As humans we are diurnal creatures, meaning we are meant to be awake during the day being active, thinking and moving. During the night, we are meant to be sleeping, resting and, recovering. Anything that is consumed other than water basically starts your circadian internal clock/internal response. Anything that is processed by your liver other than water activates these enzymes. Once they are activated, your body is on a 12-hour clock and begin to metabolize things like glucose and fatty acids efficiently and optimally.

FASTING AND HUNGER:

Before addressing hunger, it is important to distinguish the difference between physical hunger and emotional hunger. I've said it before and I'll say it again: We've been conditioned in our society to eat simply because we think we are supposed to eat. If you do something long enough, you'll develop a habit and start accepting this as gospel. I'm here to tell you to start questioning everything you read and hear, including this text right here. Digest the information and apply it. Then, try it again and figure out what works well and doesn't work well. If you think that way, you'll always improve.

CHARACTERISTICS OF PHYSICAL HUNGER:

If you're really hungry, it hits you steadily and gradually.

Any type of food can satisfy true hunger. Think about it: Have you ever been on a trip or in a place where you couldn't eat any food for a good amount of time? A friend might have some food you normally would hate. But you're starving, so you happily accept it and actually enjoy it. If you've ever been camping, I think you'll agree that food always tastes better. This is because you are more likely physically hungry instead of 'thinking' you're hungry.

When you're full, you'll stop eating. Let's say you sat down and consumed a big-ass healthy meal of chicken breast, broccoli, brown rice, and cauliflower. When you do this, chances are you'll stop eating once you're truly full. If you don't have any junk food in the house, you're most likely going to be satisfied with the healthy meal and call it a night.

When you're physically full, you're satisfied. You feel good about yourself and don't feel guilty about the meal you just ate.

EMOTIONAL EATING:

True hunger doesn't hit you suddenly like emotional hunger does. You're at work, concentrating on drafting an email to a client. Suddenly, a co-worker walks in with a giant cake for Tom's birthday celebration you forgot about. As you walk out of your office, your pupils dilate and your stomach growls while you begin thinking about how good that cake probably tastes. You weren't hungry at all until that damn cake walked its way into your life. Folks… This is emotional hunger at its finest!

Emotional hunger creates cravings. These cravings are usually specific foods that contain that awesome combo we all love: Fat + Sugar! It can even be sugar by itself. Foods like pizza, ice-cream, chocolate, peanut butter, donuts, cake, and everything else you can think of are great examples of food that most folks will have emotional hunger cravings for.

When you're emotionally full, you usually feel guilty right after swallowing the last morsel of food. Of course you feel guilty. You over-ate, and you know you overate. Your stomach feels like shit and you might not even be able to lay down without feeling uncomfortable and you'll probably have difficulty sleeping.

Having a basic understanding of true hunger compared to emotional hunger can be very beneficial for you.

WHAT TO INCLUDE DURING FASTING:

MINERALS

When fasting, your body is breaking down dead cells and waste and converting it to usable energy. During this stage of cell-cleansing and detoxification, sodium can help create a better environment for your cells.

If you are able to efficiently balance your mineral levels, an isotonic environment will be created for your cells so they have enough sodium to draw in additional water to expand and become permeable, allowing more liquids to pass through it. Think of this like a revolving door that allows nutrients and toxins to flow in and out. Creating the best environment for detoxification is one of the most important parts of controlled fasting. Yet, most forget about it.

Magnesium is crucial for digestion, muscle contraction, and nerve health.

Potassium is great for cardiovascular health and sustaining vigorous blood-pressure levels. If you're deficient in potassium levels, you will tend to feel tired and run down. However, if you include enough sodium in your diet, you won't have to worry about potassium because it's sodium sparing. So, if you get enough sodium in your diet when you fast, you won't need to worry about potassium.

This is why I believe pink Himalayan sea salt is the perfect addition to any fasting regimen.

THE IMPORTANCE OF HYDRATION

Drink enough water when you fast. Fasting promotes cell apoptosis: Programmed cell death and recycling. When you fast, your body isn't having to work on metabolizing food. Our body works on metabolizing itself. It recycles the cells and burns off what doesn't need to be there. If your body is working on this process, it needs water to mobilize the dead cells. When you're fasting, your body is utilizing fat as the primary source of fuel.

When this is taking place, understand that fat is where toxins build up. So, when we are burning fat in a fasted state, we are generating more toxins. If we aren't drinking enough water, we can't mobilize these toxins through the liver and to eliminate them. If you aren't optimally hydrated, fasting can actually stall your progress and keep you unhealthy.

So, remember to drink that H2O! Personally, I aim for 1 gallon per day.

You now understand the basics of nutrition. You now understand what fasting is and how it works. If you don't, revisit Chapter One and read it again. Now, we're going to show you how to do this shit, so you can start slaying your goals as fast as humanly possible.

WHAT TO AVOID DURING FASTING:

SWEETENERS AND ARTIFICIAL FLAVORS

Throughout my life, I've experimented with many different sweeteners and artificial flavors. There are many different products out there these days that include a lot of both. When I started competing in fitness competitions, I was in a calorie deficit, so adding no-calorie sweetness proved to be very beneficial at first. I thought, "Hey, I can add some non-calorie sweeteners in with my boring, bland, whole-foods to maximize the taste while saving myself a ton of calories! Awesome!" Well, it wasn't as awesome as I thought. For example, I experimented with different protein bars, protein powders, and other drink sweeteners. While it tasted great, I started noticing water retention and just didn't feel as great as I did before. Even as I was getting leaner, I didn't feel like it. I also noticed myself passing gas. No one wants that, especially your significant other! Haha! As soon as I started limiting my intake of artificial shit, I'd look and feel a hell of a lot leaner.

Here's the rub on artificial sweeteners during fasting. Before I go into this portion, understand this portion is only my opinion. I'm not going to go crazy with the science for this side of it because this reflects on my own personal experience, so it's anecdotal. In my opinion, I feel that taking in a lot of artificial sweeteners during a fast won't help you get the results you are aspiring for.

When you drink a few Diet Pepsis and add in a grip load of Splenda packets, your body doesn't know what the hell to do with these empty calories. It thinks it's a calorie, so it begins trying to process it like a calorie by providing you with an insulin spike. Recall earlier: When you eat food, your blood sugar rises and your pancreas signals cells to release insulin into your bloodstream to allow sugar to be converted to energy. When you eat a bunch of artificial sweeteners, you are just teasing your body with bullshit. To me, this isn't optimal for you or your results. You want to do everything you can to stabilize blood sugar and give your body the best fuel to get the best results.

My recommendation is to stay away from artificial sweeteners and colors or limit them as much as possible, especially during your time-restricted eating windows. Personally, I'll limit their intake by keeping them to a minimum. I don't limit them completely but do my best. And my results have been amazing. The point is to make you aware and give you the information and allow you to move forward for the best results.

CHAPTER SUMMARY

Controlled fasting is eating little to no food during the day. While you are allowed to consume calories, with controlled fasting, you are allowed to have some calories during the day if you are absolutely starving and need to curb your hunger

When you consume anything that isn't water during your periods of time restricted eating, you're technically breaking your fast. However, we aren't employing a water fast. In the fasting plan, we are using controlled fasting.

Understand: Being able to differentiate real hunger from emotional hunger will put you in a better position to make your fasted periods more successful.

Include minerals like pink Himalayan sea salt during your periods of time restricted eating It can create a better environment for your cells during the stage of cell cleansing and detoxification.

Make sure you drink a lot of water when you fast so you can mobilize toxins through your liver to eliminate them.

Try to limit the intake of artificial sweeteners and colors during your fasts.

CHAPTER 7. THE PRIMER PHASE

"No man has the right to be an amateur in the matter of physical training. It is a shame for a man to grow old without seeing the beauty and strength of which his body is capable."
- Socrates

Controlled fasting isn't a diet. It's more of a pattern of eating. Many folks call it 'time-restricted eating'. You will still eat the same calories. We will be changing when you eat, not what you eat. As we discussed previously, controlled fasting is eating little to no food. During this phase, you will be eating little to no food during the controlled fasting window followed by the consumption of normal meals in the afternoon.

If you haven't fasted before, it's a good idea to ease into fasting for the first week by making small adjustments. I call this first week: 'The Primer Week'. During this week, you'll be fasting for at least 12-hours. For most people, this means you'll skip your first meal at breakfast and you won't start eating until lunchtime.

If you work night shifts, try having your last meal before bed and, when waking up, ensure that a total of 12-hours have passed between your last meal and the time you resume eating the following day.

HERE'S HOW YOU DO IT:

Most people start their week on Monday, so we'll use this day as an example. On Sunday evening, you'll have your last meal and go to bed as normal. On Monday morning, wake up and drink 24-ounces of room temperature water with one teaspoon of pink Himalayan sea salt. These days, our water and food are stripped of the nutrients and minerals our bodies need to function optimally. Pink Himalayan sea salt contains 84 different kick-ass minerals and electrolytes. When we sleep for 6-9 hours during the night, we often wake up dehydrated and deficient in minerals and electrolytes.

The room temperature is said to aid the digestion and absorption of the minerals found in the sea salt. This small addition to your day can really supercharge your morning. If you want to spruce up the taste, feel free to add fresh lemon or lime to your water. I also like to add 1-scoop of Kaged Muscle-Hydra Charge to my morning drink. This supplement is not required for the program, but I do recommend it due to its hydration benefits. Keep in mind I've suggested to limit the intake of artificial sweeteners. Hydra-charge does contain sucralose, but I love that it's enhanced with stevia, which is preferable, especially on this program.

If you're interested in learning more about this, check out the 'Supplements' section in the 'Resources' chapter.

If you are a coffee drinker, I also recommend waiting for at least 1-hour after waking up to consume your coffee. So, if you wake up at 8:00 am, drink your mineral water and get your coffee to go, waiting to consume it until 9:00 am. You are allowed to have 1-2 small servings of cream in your coffee. And when I say cream, I mean half and half or something similar. You are not allowed to have any sugary-flavored creamers or any sugar-free creamers either. Basically, you are allowed to have a small amount of fat in your coffee and nothing more.

If you are hungry during the mid-morning, try having a carbonated beverage, like La-Croix or Perrier. These drinks can help reduce your hunger cravings. Make sure you consume drinks that have zero calories and zero sweeteners. The drinks mentioned above are perfect examples.

HOW YOU BREAK YOUR FAST: "THE FAST BREAK"

So, you've lasted until noon for the first day of controlled fasting. Congratulations if you've made it here! Now, it's time to break the fast. The way you beak your fast is very important. Your body is primed for nutrient uptake just as a high-performance race car. When the high-performance car runs out of fuel, you always make sure you use the high-octane fuel (best fuel) to replenish what the car has used, right? Your body is no different. The quality of the fuel will mean the difference in performance immediately and especially over time.

Before you start eating, take this 'fast break' shake. It's simple, fast, and I believe it's very beneficial for setting you up for success and ideal for improved overall health.

THERE ARE TWO DIFFERENT WAYS YOU CAN EMPLOY THE FAST BREAK.

1. Mix everything up in a small blender and knock it back.

2. Take the shot of apple cider separately. (This is my preferred way.)

INGREDIENT 1: SPRING WATER (OR FILTERED WATER)

Water will serve two purposes: Aiding digestion and contributing to your satiety. Water lubricates your joints, cushions your spinal cord, brain, and connective tissue, flushes body waste, helps maintain healthy blood pressure, etc. It also helps give you a feeling of fullness. Water fills your gut and you'll be less hungry. The less hungry you are, the easier it is to stay on point during all periods of time-restricted eating periods and controlled fasting periods. Remember: No diet, no matter how good it is, will cease to defy the physiological nature of the body. You have to create a calorie deficit if you want to burn fat.

Dose: 24 oz or 3/4 L

INGREDIENT 2: 1/8 TSP OF PINK HIMALAYAN SEA SALT

We've discussed the benefits of pink Himalayan sea salt already, so no need to go in-depth here. However, it's great for breaking your fast due to the mineral content you're replacing in your body.

Dose: 1/4 tsp

INGREDIENT 3: LEMON WATER

I believe lemons are awesome because they contain some great ingredients:

Hesperidin: A bioflavonoid that may help blood vessels function better. It may also reduce inflammation.

Citric acid: An antioxidant that protects the body from damaging free radicals.

Diosmin: Helpful for treating various disorders of blood vessels and protects against liver toxicity.

Eriocitrin: This is one of the plan pigments that gives lemons their color and is useful for it's lipid-lowering properties in liver cells. And if you can increase your chances of preventing heart disease, I'm all for it.

 Pectin: A form of soluble fiber that's been shown to help with high cholesterol, high triglycerides, and prevent cancer of the colon and prostate.

Good sources of soluble fiber can help improve gut health, aid digestion, and keep blood sugar stable. This can help with weight loss, overall health, and I believe it serves as a perfect primer for breaking your fast.

Dose: 1 tbsp juice or 1/2 lemon, blended

(Some guys recommend only consuming the lemon juice and that's okay. You are certainly welcome to do this. However, consuming the pulp of the lemon is what provides you many of the added benefits.)

INGREDIENT 4: APPLE CIDER VINEGAR

Apple cider vinegar can help stimulate the digestive system without releasing insulin. It improves overall health, helps eliminate shitty bacteria, and balances healthy levels of pH in your stomach. It even stabilizes your blood sugar levels! You want to consume something that primes the pump, so you'll be in the perfect place to absorb all the good fuel you're about to consume—and apple cider vinegar is a hell of a solution!

Dose: 1 tsp

(OPTIONAL) INGREDIENT 5: KAGED MUSCLE HYDRA CHARGE

Hydra Charge is one of my favorite supplements because it tastes so damn good. To me, it makes water more enjoyable to drink. When I like the taste of something, obviously I'm going to be inclined to drink more of it. Hydra Charge contains 5 essential electrolytes from coconut water, taurine, and SPECTRA, designed to support antioxidant potential. The reason I'm recommending it here is because of the aided hydration qualities and I believe it provides a great taste. However, you certainly are not required to use it.

Dose: 1 scoop

As I stated above, there are two ways you can do The Fast Break. I'll go more in depth here:

Method 1: Mix it all up in a blender (and take a shot of apple cider vinegar separately).

Here's how I do it: I add the water, salt, lemon, and Hydra Charge to a small blender (I have a Ninja Blender and, if you're curious, here's a link for where you can find one like I use:

https://amzn.to/2PgGT2p

I'll blend it for 20-30 seconds with a few cubes of ice. After it's done, I'll get some apple cider vinegar out, take it like a shot of tequila, and chase it with my blended shake.

Method 2: Mix everything up and drink it all together. (This is not my preferred way because apple cider vinegar has such a strong taste to me—I feel like it makes the whole shake much tougher to choke down. Kris does it this way, though. So, if you're tough as he is, go for this option!)

That's The Fast Break in its entirety. Most people consume this in a shake as do I. These steps might sound like a pain in the ass, especially because you have to blend the lemon. However, it's doable and I really think it helps with everything you're doing!

After you drink your 'fast break' shake, it's time to eat!

The order of the types of food you eat are important. Below, please find the order in which you're supposed to consume different kinds of food. Trust me, it's less complicated than you think.

ORDER OF FOOD TO BE EATEN:

1: Raw vegetables.

2: Cooked vegetables.

3: Protein.

4: Carbohydrates or fat.

As we already said, you've fasted for 12-hours and your body is primed and ready for nutrient uptake. In this fasted state, your body is like a sponge ready to ingest and utilize any fuel you give it. So choosing the appropriate fuel is of extreme importance for the following reasons:

1: Raw vegetables usually have the most nutrients compared to other foods. Get these in first and you'll notice improved energy, strength, and overall well-being. Your digestive system will act fast to break down the nutrients and turn it into usable energy.

2: Raw vegetables usually contain high amounts of fiber. Fiber not only aids in digestion but it also provides you a feeling of satiety (feeling of fullness). When you're trying to lose fat, remember you need to create a calorie deficit—you have to eat less than your body burns. When you eat less, you're almost always going to experience a sense of increased hunger. When you're hungry all the time, you obviously want to eat all the time. When you eat all the time, you're going to gain more weight/body fat. Eating more fiber in your diet makes you feel full and you'll be less likely to eat more food this way.

3: Protein is required to build muscle. Protein is also healthy for tendons, organs, skin and nails. It serves many important functions and helps stabilize your blood sugar. It's also converted to blood glucose more slowly than carbohydrates. This is an important reason why you want to include protein in your meals.

4: When most people think of fat, they think eating it will make them fat. On the contrary, including fat in your diet is another great way to stabilize your blood sugar. In fact, including fat, protein and fiber in your meals will lower the glycemic index of the foods you eat. It will help you feel fuller for longer.

Here's an example of how I break my fast. After the 'fast break' shake, I'll prepare a salad consisting of the following ingredients:

4-6 oz of grilled chicken
Baby spinach
Romaine
Arugula
Red onion
Green onion
Sliced red bell pepper
Sliced cucumber
Carrots

Celery
Tomatoes
Sugar snap peas

I also throw in a small amount* of salad topping ingredients like:

Bacon bits
Wonton strips
Tortilla strips
Dried cranberries
etc.

*For these, I use a minimal amount, which adds a lot of taste and makes for one epic salad. For dressing, I use vinegar or balsamic vinegar. Also, a note on seasonings: I don't skimp on salt, either—I like salt and pepper, as well as seasoned salt.

RULE: For meals in the afternoon and evening, remember the following: Always drink 1 glass of water and eat veggies with each meal.

What types of meals can you eat? Just about anything you would normally eat. Just make sure you add veggies. Try to eat healthy, of course. This means try to avoid eating out and stay away from fast food restaurants.

For your eating window, try and space your meals a few hours apart. That being said, you can have as many meals during this time as you like. If you break your fast at noon, your next meals will be 3:00 pm and 6:00 pm respectively. Personally, I prefer to have 2 or 3 meals evenly spaced apart during my feeding window during this Primer Phase. I like doing it this way due to its simplicity and convenience.

When you are done eating for the day, try to make sure this last meal is consumed within 2-hours before bedtime. Doing this allows your digestive system ample time to work on processing your food and passing it to your small intestine. So, by the time you jump in bed, your body has had the chance to process the last meal of the day. The idea to stop eating 2-hours before bedtime also relates to our circadian rhythm. In the evening, our body starts preparing for rest by producing melatonin, a sleep hormone. In a recent study, 110 college students aged 18-22 were observed for a 30-day sleep-wake period.

"Researchers assessed meals, calories consumed, and their timing against sleep, activity and body fat. They noticed that for individuals with higher body fat, the midpoint of all the calories they consumed for the day was later than for leaner people, and 1 hour closer to the onset of melatonin release" (Kinsey & Ormsbee 2015).

There are various studies showing people who eat immediately before bed have a higher probability of gaining more weight (Reid, Baron, & Zee, 2014) (Spaeth, Dinges, & Goel, 2013).

The practice of avoiding food at least 2-hours before bedtime gives our digestive system a break and serves our circadian rhythm more positively. When it's time to sleep, you want to take advantage of the most optimal strategy designed to get the best bang for the buck. Interfering with your circadian rhythm isn't your best bet.

[The primer week should give you basic understanding of fasting and how to deal with hunger and satiety. Knowing your body and how it responds to different instances will give you a better frame of reference as it relates to fasting and health in general.]

PUTTING IT ALL TOGETHER

Rules of the Primer Phase:

•	The goal is to fast 12-hours each day. (For most people, you usually won't start eating until 12:00 pm.)

•	During your controlled fasting period, try to make it through without eating anything. However, you are allowed to have some calories during this time. For example, you can have trace amounts of creamer with your coffee and/or a pre-workout supplement if you work out in the morning.

•	Consume the 'fast break' shake before you start eating your first meal.

•	For your first meal after the fast break, try eating a salad and include as many different textures and colors as possible.

For other meals:

•	Drink 1 glass of water with each meal.

•	Eat veggies with each meal.

•	Try and space meals a few hours apart if you can.

- Try and finish eating your final meal of the day 2-hours before bedtime.

CHAPTER 8. THE ACCLIMATION PHASE

"Success is not final, failure is not fatal: it is the courage to
continue that counts. "
-Winston Churchill

During this phase of controlled fasting, small adjustments
will be made to your time-restricted eating schedule and
help you gain an even better understanding of how fasting
works. FYI: This will continue to get a little more difficult
during each phase. Just remember: You're not depriving
yourself of anything. For the most part, you aren't changing
WHAT you eat, you are simply changing WHEN you eat.

Do you think you're ready? If so, let's get into it.

This week, you aren't going to start eating until the
afternoon. Have I scared you yet? Don't worry—it's not that
bad. We are going to follow the similar rules as The Primer
Phase with a few modifications.

Day One - Day Three: Begin eating your first meal in the mid-
afternoon. In a sense, you're going to skip breakfast and
lunch. Drink 20 oz of water immediately after you wake up in
the morning. It's okay to have coffee with trace amounts of
cream. If you are starving and just can't take it, it's okay to
have a whey protein shake in the mid-morning (example:
Kaged Muscle Re-Kaged).

(Remember, we are implementing a 'controlled fasting' protocol. This means we are eating little to no food during the under-eating phase. During a water fast, you wouldn't eat anything. The only thing you'd consume is water. I bring this up because it's a very popular question.)

Try to drink as much water as you can during the day. Once you make it to your mid-afternoon feeding window, you're going to begin your meal with a salad, just as you did during The Primer Phase. Try to include as many different colors and textures as possible. It's okay to include any meat you like (i.e. whole eggs, chicken, steak, fish, etc.).

For protein amounts, follow the following suggestion: For males, aim for a 6-8 oz serving of protein. For females, aim for a 4-5 oz serving of protein. You are free to eat more protein if you like, just make sure you eat at least 6 oz per serving for men and 4 oz per serving for women.

For the meal or two following, drink 20 oz of water before you eat. Include veggies as well. Stop eating your last meal of the day at least 2-hours before bedtime.

RULES OF THE ACCLIMATION PHASE:

Don't start eating until mid-afternoon (preferably 2:00 pm or 3:00 pm).

Drink a glass of water with each meal.

First meal: Eat a salad and include as many different colors and textures as possible.

All other meals: Eat the foods you'd normally eat BUT include veggies.

Protein in each meal: Eat at least 6 oz per serving for men and 4 oz per serving for women.

Drink 1 glass of water with each meal (and it's suggested that you try and drink around 1 gallon of water by end the day).

Eat veggies with each meal.

Try and space meals a few hours apart if you can.

Try and finish eating your final meal of the day 2-hours before bedtime.

That's it! Really, the only difference between The Primer Phase and The Acclimation Phase is adjusting the periods of time-restricted eating windows. The theories taught in The Fasting Plan are simple, but they aren't necessarily easy. The goal in developing this program has and always will be: To get you positive results in your health and appearance that stay with you throughout your life! We are about to change who we are for who we will become! ▢

Chapter 9: The Fasting Plan For Fat Burning

> "To be successful, you must be willing to, at any moment , sacrifice who you are for what you will become."
> -Eric Thomas

Once you've completed The Primer Phase and The Acclimation Phase, you're now ready to begin The Fat Burning Protocol. You're used to fasting now and have a good idea of what to expect. We will start with a cycle of controlled fasting combining the following forms:

22/2 or 20/4 Controlled Intermittent Fasting

16/8 Controlled Intermittent Fasting

Day One - Day Four: We will be implementing the 22/2 Controlled Intermittent Fasting technique. Since most people begin their week on Monday, we will start with this day. However, it doesn't matter which day of the week you begin the Fat Burning Protocol. Remember that controlled fasting consists of eating little to no calories during the day. I've found that people work better when they have specific guidelines, so the rules are as follows:

RULE 1: *EAT NO MORE THAN 200 CALORIES DURING THE CONTROLLED FASTING WINDOW.*

RULE 2: *YOU MUST DRINK ¾ - 1 GALLON OF WATER DURING THE CONTROLLED FASTING WINDOW.*

*Follow these rules 100 percent. No questions. No exceptions.

Here's how the days will break down:

In our example, the program starts on Monday. You'll have your last meal on Sunday night. On Monday morning, you'll wake up and begin your controlled fasting time period. The plan is to fast all day by eating little to no food. But, if you are starving, you are allowed to have some veggies. I also prefer to have trace amounts of creamer in my coffee because I enjoy it.

YOUR DAY WILL START LIKE THIS:

5:30 am: Wake up and drink the 'fast break' shake consisting of:

20-24 oz of spring water

1/4 lemon

1/8 tsp of pink Himalayan sea salt

Optional

1 scoop of Kaged Muscle Hydra Charge

1 scoop of Kaged Muscle L-Glutamine

1 tsp of organic turmeric

5:45 am: Activity

Studies have shown that getting your blood moving in the morning upon waking up can improve your thermogenesis during the day. Here is a very brief workout that will get your heart rate up and will set you up for success. Try the following routine which should only take you 5-10 minutes. If you can't perform 100 push-ups in a row, complete as many as you can and rest for 15-30 seconds. Keep pushing out reps and resting until you complete all 100 reps.

1-   100 Push-ups

2-   20 Burpees

3-   3 Sets of 30 crunches with bands

8:00 am: Start working and have more water

9:00 am: Coffee with cream

10:30 am: Sparkling water

*2:00 pm: Small veggie meal

If you are starving your ass off and don't think you'll make it until the evening 'feeding window", go ahead and eat a vegetable tray with a low-fat ranch dressing or hummus. If you can make it without eating this meal, that is optimal. A decent time to do this is anywhere from 12:00 pm to 2:00 pm.

An example is:

1 sliced red bell pepper
100g of sugar snap peas
10 carrots
50g of cauliflower
1 sliced tomato

5:00 PM: Consume Pre-Workout with 20-24 oz of water

5:30 PM: Workout

7-7:30 PM: Time to eat

IF YOU WORK OUT IN THE AM:

If you work out in the morning, go ahead and hit the gym. If you take a pre-workout, go ahead and drink it with another 20 oz of water 30-minutes before hitting the gym. I recommend Pre-Kaged by Kaged Muscle Supplements. Since this program implements controlled fasting instead of water fasting, you will have little to no food during your fasting (time-restricted eating) window. This is why you can have pre-workout supplements and/or small amounts of certain foods and drinks.

After you've finished the workout, drink more water. For taste, you can add lemon to it.

If you are absolutely starving after the gym, you are allowed to have a small whey protein shake with water (no more than 30g of protein). If you can make it without the whey protein, that is optimal. Having protein powder isn't necessary in my opinion. Since our goal in this chapter is to burn as much fat as possible, we are going to do everything we can to maximize our body's dependence on using stored fat as energy instead of glycogen. The lower amount of food we ingest will also help promote autophagy (cell-cleansing) and aid in helping improve our insulin sensitivity.

The rest of the day, the point is to avoid food and focus on work. This is your time-restricted eating window. During the morning hours, you will be the hungriest—understanding this, you can have coffee with trace amounts of creamer (half and half is okay but stay away from sugar-free creamers and other sugary creamers).

You can also have sparkling water beverages, like Perrier, Pellegrino, and La-Croix. These are great because they help curb your hunger and are pretty tasty.

The above are only examples. You can also combine these into a small salad. The idea is to eat a good amount of veggies you enjoy until you have a full feeling—but try not to overdo it. Eating veggies or having whey protein won't necessarily affect your progress, but if you get to the point where you don't need any food, you will have more control over your body and mind. This will help you turn this program into a way of life. If you can stick to this, guess what? You're going to get lean and stay lean all year long as I have.

THE FEEDING WINDOW:

After you've fasted during the day, it's time to finally eat. This is where the fun begins. Usually, I choose to eat around 6:00 pm or 7:00 pm if I've worked out in the morning. I don't set a specific time. However, I focus on trying to fast as long as possible during the day to give my body a chance to burn fat and detoxify. Usually, the time-restricted period of eating lasts around 20-22 hours. (Hence the names '20/4' and '22/2'.)

For The Fasting Plan, every time you break your fast, you are instructed to perform The Fast Break (discussed in Chapter 6).

After you employ The Fast Break, the order of foods to be eaten is important. Refer to the directions below.

ORDER OF FOOD TO BE EATEN:

You've fasted for most of the day and your body is primed and ready for nutrient uptake. In this fasted state, your body is like a sponge ready to ingest and utilize any fuel you give it. So, choosing the appropriate fuel is of extreme importance. Here's the order of food to be eaten:

1: Raw vegetables

2: Cooked vegetables

3: Protein

4: Carbohydrates or fat

Eating food in the order described above will give you better results because you'll eat the nutrient-dense foods first, giving your body a higher grade of fuel. The fiber from the nutrient-dense foods will also give you a better feeling of satiety. The fuller you are, the less likely you are to overeat. See what I'm getting at here? Magic pills aren't the answer and they don't exist anyway.

The following is an example of how I break my fast. First, I'll have the 'fast break' shake. Then, I'll make myself the following salad:

1c spinach
1c romaine lettuce
1 sliced bell pepper
half cucumber
1/4c corn
1/2c blueberries
1/4c cherry tomatoes
vinegar for dressing

While I'm eating my salad, I'll grill some asparagus on the barbecue, adding some non-fat cooking spray and garlic salt.

For protein, I'll grill some flank steak or petite sirloin. I prefer cuts that are lean. Sometimes I'll have rice with the steak and other times I'll have a baked potato (white or sweet potato).

Above is only an example. The main goal is to eat veggies first and follow it up with protein and carbs. Experiment with the food that you enjoy the most. Refer to the list of nutrient-dense foods at the beginning of this chapter if you need more ideas. I've also included recipes at the end of the book in the 'References' section for your convenience.

Eat your dinner and enjoy yourself. This is the time to eat as much as you like with no guilt. Eating food in that order is optimal because it fuels your body with fiber, vitamins, and other great stuff before you eat everything else. In a fasted state, your body is in a perfect position to partition nutrients into your muscle as opposed to fat.

Pay attention to your hunger and thirst as you eat. Once you become thirstier than you are hungry, stop eating for 20-30 minutes. I have to thank Ori Hofmekler for this great tip. In his book 'The Warrior Diet', he recommends the same. However, he likes to wait 10-15 minutes in this state and I prefer to wait longer to give my body a better chance to digest what I've eaten.

Above is how the 20-4 fast is done. You will do the 20-4 fast Monday through Thursday (or 4-days per week if you start on a different day).

On Friday and Saturday, you will employ a 16-8 fast. Try to schedule your eating window between 12:00 pm and 8:00 pm if you can. I've found this is the most convenient and the most effective. These days will be similar to what you did during The Primer Phase. Just remember to fast for 16-hours.

RULES FOR THE FAT BURNING PROTOCOL:

- 20/4: Fast for 20-hours; eat during a 4-hour window.

- 16/8: Fast for 16-hours; eat during an 8-hour window.

- Drink this everyday upon waking: 24 oz of room temperature water with pink Himalayan sea salt. (Optional: Add Kaged Muscle Hydra Charge for taste.)

- Wait 1-hour after waking up to consume coffee (with have trace amounts of cream if you like).

- If you're hungry in mid-morning, you can have sparkling water (a zero calorie, zero sweetener, carbonated beverage).

- Eat no more than 200 calories during your fasting period.

- Consume the 'fast break' shake before you start eating your first meal.

- For your first meal after The Fast Break, try eating a salad and include as many different textures and colors as possible.

For other meals:

- Drink 1 glass of water with each meal.

- Eat veggies with each meal.

- Try and space meals a few hours apart if you can.

- Try and finish eating your final meal of the day 2-hours before bedtime.

On the last day of the week, you'll eat as you normally would—you won't be fasting. This day will serve as a re-feed day. I like to call it a 'reset day'. Over the years of my fitness competition days, I used a lot of methods of dieting. One of my favorites was carb cycling. This simply means you'd adjust carbohydrate amounts during the week while keeping your body in a deficit to burn fat. An example would be to eat low carbs Monday through Thursday, medium amounts of carbs on Friday and Saturday, and follow it up with a high day on Sunday. This helped me burn fat and primed me for the fitness show by giving me an idea of how my body would react to higher amounts of carbs. This idea is called glycogen supercompensation.

Bodybuilders have used this form of dieting for years to burn fat and it's been very successful for them. Without going too in-depth, your body gets fuel from carbohydrates and stores them in your muscle as glycogen. This is what gives your muscles the full look. The rest is stored in your liver. When you strip yourself from carbs for long enough periods of time, your body will look flat and depleted. You'll burn high amounts of fat in this state, but you'll look and feel like shit. Since your body has been depleted, it soaks up carbs like a sponge when you reintroduce them into your diet. It's said that your body might hold as much as 2 to 2.5 times the normal amounts of glycogen. This is why they call it 'glycogen supercompensation'.

This was great when I did shows because it helped me get leaner while giving me an idea of what my body would look like after being super-compensated with glycogen. Each week, as I would get leaner, I would be able to tighten up and tweak the amount of carbs I'd need to look my best for the show.

This idea of carb cycling led me to throw around the idea of cycling the types of fasting for better results. This is how The Fasting Plan was born. Cycling the different types of fasting days, followed with a re-feed day (reset day), would provide you with a significant advantage of fat burning. The reset day has proven itself to be a great addition as well. While I haven't performed studies on this type of cycling, I have had lots of personal success with this type of fasting as well as many of my clients. I'm saying this to you because I love this stuff and I'd like you to know how I've stumbled upon this technique and I'm eager to hear your feedback. So far, the results have been incredible!

TO SUMMARIZE, THE FAT BURNING PROTOCOL WILL BREAK DOWN AS FOLLOWS:

- Monday through Thursday: 20-4 Fast

- Friday and Saturday: 16-8 Fast

- Sunday: Reset Day

- Repeat everything again the next week. I've been living this lifestyle for a longtime. It's very simple and reproducible, allowing for strong flexibility. This makes it easier to adhere to—and remember: The keys to every successful program starts with adherence.

CHAPTER 10: RESOURCES

As promised, this section includes bonus material and I've broken it down into the following sections:

FAQ for the Primer Phase

FAQ for the Acclimation Phase

Fast-Breaking Recipes

How to Control Hunger

This is just the tip of the iceberg. There will be future updates to this section. So, check it out and hit me up on social media with your feedback, suggestions, and questions!

THE FASTING PLAN FAQS

FAQ Section for The Primer Phase:

Q: What if I work nights?

A: It doesn't matter what time you work. Just skip your first meal and begin eating in the middle of 'your day'. For example, if you're a hospital worker, your day would start like this:

7 pm: Wake up

9 pm: Begin work

12 am: Assuming this is your lunchtime, you'd begin eating your first meal here. Eat your meals like normal (including The Primer Phase rules).

11 am: Assuming you'd go to bed at time, stop eating at 9 am or earlier.

Q: When do I work out during this Primer Phase?

A: It doesn't matter. Whatever time is most convenient will work.

Q: Can I drink anything else during my fasting window in the mornings?

A: Yes. You can drink coffee with small amounts of cream if you wish.

Q: If I'm seeing results with the Primer Phase, is it okay to keep doing it?

A: Of course. This week is a form of time-restricted eating and will help you get in shape. In my opinion it's perfectly fine to eat this way all the time if you wish.

Q: Can I have any other food during my fast?

A: No. For this week, we're only fasting for a few hours after we wake up. You can do this, right? It's only a few hours! Lol

Q: What about supplements? Can I have any during my fast?

A: Yes and no. During this week, you can use supplements that contain little to no calories. Pre-workouts like Kaged Muscle Pre-Kaged work great. If you lift in the am, go ahead and take a pre-workout.

Other supplements that don't contain a lot of carbs (less than 10 carbs) are okay. Examples:BCAAs (Kaged Muscle BCAA Powder, Pre-Kaged, or In-Kaged)

Intra workout products (Kaged Muscle In-Kaged)

Hydrating products (Kaged Muscle Hydra Charge)

Supplements not to take during this fasted window:

Protein powders, high-carb powders, etc.

(The idea is to keep calories low during the fasted window. Just look at the labels of products to confirm. As a rule of thumb: If it has more than 10 carbs, 10 grams of protein, or 10 grams of fat per serving, don't use it during your fasting window. You can take these types of products after you break your controlled fast.)

FAQ Section for The Acclimation Phase:

Q: I'm starving and don't think I can go this whole week waiting to eat my first meal until the afternoon. Can I go back to having my first meal in the middle of the day instead of afternoon?

A: Yes. You are still trying to get used to fasting and how your body is reacting to these new changes. If you find it too difficult to wait until the afternoon to start eating, you can go back to eating your first meal at noon. However, I'd like you to follow the rules for The Acclimation Phase for at least 3-days before you go back to eating at noon. Remember: You're feeling hunger pains because your body is not used to going this long without eating. But guess what? Your body is turning up its fat-burning capabilities and autophagy (cell cleansing). If you can follow this protocol, I am very confident you are going to love the results. You want to feel better and look better? Stay true to the plan and keep working hard. Nothing worth having is easy. You can do this!

Q: When do I work out during the Acclimation Phase?

A: It doesn't matter. Whatever time is most convenient will work.

Q: Can I drink anything else during my fasting window in the mornings?

A: Yes. You can drink coffee with small amounts of cream if you wish.

Q: Can I have any other food during my fast?

A: Yes. You can have veggies and one whey protein shake (but aim for not consuming more than 30 grams of protein). The idea is to keep your food consumption amounts small. We want to fire up your body's thermogenesis (fat burning) and improve your health. Giving your digestive system a break is the name of the game.

FAST-BREAK RECIPES:

As I say in The Fasting Plan, when you break your fast, I recommend using as many different colors and textures as possible when you're creating your meal. Ori Hofmekler also teaches this in his book "The Warrior Diet". Incorporating different tastes and textures in your food is both healthy and extremely satisfying to your taste buds. And after fasting, your body is primed to soak up any nutrient-dense food you can provide it with. You'll be more satiated, and your abs will start showing up more.

You don't have to use every single ingredient I mentioned. However, I've found that using different forms of lettuce (shredded lettuce, romaine, and spinach) helps to make the meal more interesting and enjoyable. So, most of the time, I definitely include these!

For protein, I usually use turkey and cook it over the stove with non-stick cooking spray.

The key is to use as many healthy options (nutrient-dense types of food) as you can. And feel free to add in a little of the unhealthier options like wonton strips or bacon bits. Adding small amounts of things like this will give your salad a huge bump in taste quality! You don't have to add much. Just a little will do.

CONTROLLED FASTING POWER SHAKE

Ingredients:

20 oz water
2 cups spinach or more
1 cup frozen strawberries

1 scoop Hydra Charge
3/4 scoop casein protein powder
5 g of l-glutamine
1/2 scoop whey isolate
1 scoop greens powder

Instructions:

Mix everything up in a blender. This is a lot to consume. No
doubt you might have a tough time finishing it. You should be
full once you're done with it.

HUNGER-DESTROYING FASTING SALAD

Ingredients:

Spinach
Romaine lettuce
Shredded lettuce
Carrots
Tomatoes
Reduced fat blue cheese crumbles
Celery
Bell peppers (Any color you like. I prefer red bell peppers)
Cucumbers
Season salt
Avocado
Won Ton strips
Tortilla strips
Corn
Bacon bits or cooked bacon (2 slices)
Turkey or chicken
Non-fat vinegar dressing or low-fat blue cheese dressing

Instructions

As I say in The Fasting Plan, when you break your fast, I recommend using as many different colors and textures as possible when you're creating your meal. Incorporating different tastes and textures in your food is both healthy and extremely satisfying to your taste buds. And after fasting, your body is primed to soak up any nutrient dense food you can provide it with. You'll be more satiated and your abs will start showing up more as well.

You don't have to use every single ingredient I mentioned. However, I've found that using different forms of lettuce (shredded lettuce, romaine and spinach) helps to make the meal more interested and enjoyable. So, most of the time, I definitely include these!

For protein, I usually use turkey and cook it over the stove with non-stick cooking spray.

The key is to use as many healthy options (nutrient dense types of food) as you can. And feel free to add in a little of the more unhealthy options like wonton strips or bacon bits. Adding small amounts of things like this will give your salad a huge bump in taste quality! You don't have to add much. Just a little will do.

Bad-Ass Steak Tacos

Ingredients:

Coleslaw
Flank steak
1 sweet onion
1 bunch cilantro
Lime juice

Garlic salt
Montreal Steak Seasoning
Non-Stick Cooking spray
small corn tortillas
Avocado

Instructions:

Preheat the oven on 'Broil'. Place tin foil on a cookie sheet
and coat it with non-stick cooking spray. Place the flank steak
on the pan and season with Montreal steak seasoning. Put in
oven for 8-minutes. Pull out of the oven and flip steak over
and put it back in for another 8-minutes. If you like your
steak a little more done, you can place it back in the over for
another 5-minutes. I like to make a few cuts in the center of
the steak. This lets me see how well it cooks and also makes
things go a little faster, in my opinion.

For the taco slaw, add the following ingredients into a big
salad bowl:

1 package of coleslaw
diced cilantro
1 diced sweet onion
3 tbsp of lime juice
Season with garlic salt as desired
*Mix up well

Here is the special part that most people don't think about.
Heat up a 12-inch frying pan at medium heat, coated with
non-stick cooking spray. Place 3-4 corn tortillas in the pan
and coat each side with non-stick cooking spray. Fry them
until each side is brown.

Once the steak is done, dice it up into small pieces and add to the tacos. Place some slaw over it and top it off with a slice of an avocado and garnish with a lime wedge. Sometimes, I'll dice the steak and throw it in the pan and heat up the steak a little more for a few minutes before adding it to the tacos. I also love to use hot sauce when eating these bad boys. My favorite brand to eat with these are Frank's RedHot Buffalo Wing Sauce.

FAT-SHREDDING CAULIFLOWER PIZZA

(This is one of the simplest recipes I've found. However, it took me a long time to get it right. You see, most people who try to make cauliflower pizza screw up the crust.)

Ingredients:

1 head of cauliflower (or you can buy cauliflower that is already diced up at most grocery stores these days). Alternatively, you can buy frozen cauliflower (2 x 16 oz bags). These options all work pretty much the same.

Non-Fat shredded cheese (cheddar)
Low-fat shredded mozzarella cheese
2 whole eggs
pizza seasoning
Cookie sheet
Parchment paper
Dish towel
Turkey or chicken
Garlic
Non-fat cooking spray

Instructions:

Preheat the oven to 450 degrees.

Place the head of cauliflower in a food processor or blender (I have a Ninja, so that's what I use—and it works great). Blend the cauliflower until it reaches a rice consistency. At this stage, you can heat it up in the microwave or boil it on the stove top. Both options take anywhere from 10-15 minutes.

After the cauliflower reaches a smooth texture, take it off heat and let it sit for ~5-minutes. If boiling, drain the excess water from the cauliflower.

Place the dishtowel on your counter and place the cauliflower on top. At this point, you're going to use the towel to strain the excess moisture out of the cauliflower. This is the magic step that will make your crust crispy! Try and squeeze as much moisture out of the cauliflower as you can. I am basic, so I use a dishtowel. If you have the means, feel free to use a nut milk bag instead. I'll leave a link below for your convenience.

Beat the 2 whole eggs and add them to a large bowl. Then add the cauliflower with 56 grams of non-fat cheese, 56 grams of low-fat mozzarella cheese, 1 tsp of garlic, and a few pinches of pizza seasoning. Mix everything together well. I like to do this while the cauliflower is still warm. Doing this will allow you to create a nice, pizza-dough consistency.

Place the parchment paper on the cookie sheet and spray it with non-stick cooking spray. Spread the dough onto the parchment paper evenly. I like to use my hands. Use a spatula if you like.

Cook it in the oven for 12-15 minutes or until you reach a nice, brown consistency. If you like crispier crust, cook it a little longer.

Once the crust is finished, you can garnish it with your protein, garlic salt, extra cheese, etc. Enjoy!

HIGH PROTEIN FASTING STEW

Ingredients:

2 diced tomatoes
1 diced onion
1 bell pepper
1 cup fresh corn
5 diced celery stalks
Tomato bouillon (1-2 cubes)
94%-97% lean ground beef (or turkey)
1 clove garlic chopped
1 small can on tomato paste
Chili powder
Cumin
Oregano
Salt
Cayenne
1 cup water

Instructions:

Cook the ground beef until brown on medium heat. Drain off the excess fat, and then pour in the tomato sauce, water, chili powder, cumin, oregano, salt, tomato bouillon, cayenne, and all the veggies. Stir everything together and reduce the heat too low. Simmer for about 30-minutes and stir occasionally. You may have to add more water occasionally to keep it from getting dry.

Serve with shredded non-fat cheese, chopped onions, tortilla chips, or lime wedges. Be creative and do feel free to experiment with more options.

Stir together well, cover, and then reduce the heat to low. Simmer for 1-hour, stirring occasionally. If the mixture becomes overly dry, add 1/2 cup water at a time as needed.

HOW TO CONTROL HUNGER

Before I started fasting, I thought it would make me miserable, sluggish, and energy deprived. I was scared of being hungry all the time! After all, fasting means you have to go without food, right? Once I studied fasting and started applying it, not only have I got in the best shape of my life, I've also improved my relationship with food, experienced enhanced mental clarity during work, and feel better than I ever have. In this section, you'll find a few tips and tactics I've found and used along the way. Enjoy.

3 life-saving tips to control your hunger and burn fat with fasting! If you control hunger, you control everything.

Tip #1: Understand the difference between emotional hunger and real hunger.

If you're really hungry, it hits you steadily and gradually. Any type of food can satisfy true hunger.

Think about it.

Have you ever been on a trip or in a place where you couldn't eat any food for a good amount of time? A friend might have some food you normally would hate. But you're starving, and you happily accept it and actually enjoy it. If you've ever been camping, I think you'll agree that food always tastes better. This is because you are more likely physically hungry instead of 'thinking' you're hungry.

When you're full, you'll stop eating. Let's say you sat down and consumed a big-ass healthy meal of chicken breast, broccoli, brown rice, and cauliflower.

When you do this, chances are you'll stop eating once you're truly full. If you don't have any junk food in the house, you're most likely going to be satisfied with the healthy meal and call it a night.

Tip #2: Water! The importance of proper hydration.

Drink enough water when you fast. Fasting promotes cell apoptosis: programmed cell death and recycling. When you fast, your body isn't having to work on metabolizing food. Our body works on metabolizing itself. It recycles the cells and burns off what doesn't need to be there. If your body is working on this process, it needs water to mobilize the dead cells. When you're fasting, your body is utilizing fat as the primary source of fuel.

Tip #3: Understand and apply controlled fasting approach.

In The Fasting Plan, we will be employing the controlled fasting technique. This means you will be eating 'little to no food' during the day and saving the majority of your macronutrients for the evening.

In the mornings, I add cream to my coffee. I try to last the whole day without eating any food but sometimes, I get more hungry than other days. When this happens, I'll run to the store and get a small veggie tray and dip it in hummus. Usually, this is around 2 pm in the afternoon.

This will hold me over until the evening where I will eat the majority of my food for that day. (I like breaking my fast around 7 pm.)

"But Nick! Aren't you breaking your fast?" If you are doing a water fast, yes. But we are using controlled fasting, remember?

The veggies are great because they contain a lot of fiber and a good amount of nutrients. The fiber will help tide me over until that evening meal and I still get to experience the benefits of controlled fasting.

Adding some veggies to my diet here and there will help make this program easier to stick to!

Adherence is a very important factor for any successful program. After all, you won't stick to something if you hate it, right?

MORE TIPS ON HUNGER AND HOW TO CONTROL IT.

The most common concern that people have about fasting is that their hunger will overwhelm them and make them prone to overeating.

We are human, and hunger is a natural phenomenon. We have to eat to survive but we don't have to indulge in overeating to survive. We, as humans, are conditioned to constantly thinking about food. Imagine you are going to the movies, but wait a second—how can you watch a movie without popcorn and soda? See, even if you just had dinner, the craving for popcorn is too much to resist.

Habit breaking is the first step to controlling hunger while fasting. For example, if you have a habit of munching while watching TV, try shifting from snacks like chips and nuts to drinking water or herbal tea. And then slowly quitting this habit altogether.

Find motivation to fast. This is one of the key factors that affects the difficulty you face while fasting. If your motivation to commit to your diet is stronger than your hunger, then things will slowly get easier for you.

When you feel tired and have low energy, you'll start to think that it might be due to the fact that you're fasting and haven't eaten all day. But in reality, it could just be the fact that you haven't had enough sleep.

Distract yourself from hunger. Because most eat away their boredom, please don't be like that. Try going for a walk, watching a movie, or simply hanging out with your family to distract yourself from your attention seeking growling stomach.

The thing that helps distract most from hunger is talking to a friend. Pick up your phone, call a friend, and, believe me, talking fills up the belly like nothing else.

Try to eat healthy and nutrition-packed food in the non-fasting period. Try not to let your palate take you on an eight-course meal of overindulgence. Maintain proper portions of fruits, vegetables, and proteins. Drink herbal tea to help soothe and revitalize the body from within.

These are a few tried and tested tips for fighting hunger while fasting. I hope they help make you day easier.

Cheers to striving towards health and fitness!

SUPPLEMENTS THAT HELP WITH HUNGER:

Caffeine:

There isn't enough that can be said about the great benefits of caffeine. It helps me with clarity, assists with thermogenesis (fat burning), and makes me focus. But guess what else it does? Yep, it acts an appetite suppressant.

Coffee:

When fasting, I love to drink a few cups of coffee during the day. I add cream to it as well. Remember, this is controlled fasting not water fasting.

Green Tea:

This is another one of my favorites. It tastes great and helps give me a full feeling. Normally, I stick with coffee as my go-to. Green tea is a nice change of pace though. Research shows it also helps with thermogenesis too. Since we're trying to burn fat here, this is definitely an added benefit.

PurCaf:

Organic caffeine from Kaged Muscle. These little capsules have saved my life a few times. I feel that the natural, organic caffeine provides me with a steady amount of energy throughout the day. I like to use this instead of energy drinks for one simple reason: There are many different forms of caffeine and some are better than others. Some energy drinks I've tried give me tons of energy right off the bat, but then hit a wall soon thereafter. This idea is similar to eating a candy bar. It gives you a quick insulin spike of energy and then you crash. I hate that.

Sparkling Water:

I love using this and drink it just about every day. Using something that's carbonated gives me a different taste and allows me to enjoy another option that is zero calories.

The Fasting Plan Quick Start Guide: How To Use Fasting To Burn Fat ASAP

This Fat Burning Protocol combines what I feel are the most superior forms of fasting in the best ways to product optimal results. The goal is to get lean and stay lean all year long. This doesn't matter if you're staying in town and are able to stay on a consistent work schedule or if you're traveling seventy-five percent of the time. The fasting plan will allow you to control your life by putting you in the driver's seat. You will be able to start controlling your environment instead of getting controlled by it.

In this quick-start guide, we will cover the most popular form of the fasting plan to help you start burning fat fast. You're new to this program and you might be new to fasting. Either way, the goal of the fasting plan is to teach you how to learn the fasting techniques that will give you amazing results that will stay with you for life. Here's how it's going to work:

Step 1: The Primer Phase

What it is: This week-long period of time is designed to introduce you to fasting by slowly priming your body for what's to come. You will introduce time-restricted eating into your routine to teach you what it feels like to extend the controlled fasting periods.

STEP 2: THE ACCLIMATION PHASE

What it is: Right after you complete the Primer Phase, you will continue with the Acclimation Phase. During this time, we will continue to tweak the time-restricted eating periods, help you improve the ways you deal with hunger, learn how to periodize your fasting segments, and develop a fast-breaking strategy.

STEP 3: THE FAT-BURNING FASTING PLAN

What it is: Once you complete the Primer Phase and the Acclimation Phase, you are ready to jump in 100 percent and experience the heart and soul of the full fasting program.

The Primer and Acclimation Phases are designed to, not only introduce you to the fasting program, but more importantly, to periodize your time-restricted eating periods, so you can teach yourself to be more efficient at burning calories. By doing everything in order, your chances of success will be much higher and you're more likely to stick to this long-term. And if long-term results are what you're after, make sure you complete these phases. Think of this program like a recipe for baking a cake. If you pre-heat the oven and perform action steps in the order they are recommended, you'll have a perfect, mouth-watering dessert to offer friends and family. If you don't follow the instructions, or screw up the order of tasks, all sorts of things could go wrong. The cake might not rise. It could have a terrible consistency. Or, even worse, you end up with a burnt cake that leaves an after smell in your house for a week!

You get my point, right? Good. And just so you know, the way I write might seem repetitive at times. I won't apologize for that because I want to hammer these points home, so they become permanent with you. The more these principles are engrained in your psyche, the more successful I believe you'll be. Ahem. Back to the program!

If you follow the instructions for the fasting program correctly, you'll start to understand what true hunger is and is not. You'll start learning to understand your body more in-depth and this will help you improve your body composition and overall health in a durable way that will last your lifetime!

THE PRIMER PHASE

Controlled fasting isn't a diet. It's more of a pattern of eating. Many folks call it 'time-restricted eating'. You will still eat the same calories. We will be changing when you eat, not what you eat. As we discussed previously, controlled fasting is eating little to no food. During this phase, you will be eating little to no food during the controlled fasting window followed by the consumption of normal meals in the afternoon.

If you haven't fasted before, it's a good idea to ease into fasting for the first week by making small adjustments. I call this first week: 'The Primer Week'. During this week, you'll be fasting for at least 12-hours. For most people, this means you'll skip your first meal at breakfast and you won't start eating until lunchtime.

If you work night shifts, try having your last meal before bed and, when waking up, ensure that a total of 12-hours have passed between your last meal and the time you resume eating the following day.

Here's how you do it:

Most people start their week on Monday, so we'll use this day as an example. On Sunday evening, you'll have your last meal and go to bed as normal. On Monday morning, wake up and drink 24-ounces of room temperature water with one teaspoon of pink Himalayan sea salt. These days, our water and food are stripped of the nutrients and minerals our body's need to function optimally. Pink Himalayan sea salt contains 84 different kick-ass minerals and electrolytes. When we sleep for 6-9 hours during the night, we often wake up dehydrated and deficient in minerals and electrolytes. The room temperature is said to aid the digestion and absorption of the minerals found in the sea salt. This small addition to your day can really supercharge your morning. If you want to spruce up the taste, feel free to add fresh lemon or lime to your water. I also like to add 1-scoop of Kaged Muscle Hydra Charge to my morning drink. This supplement is not required for the program, but I do recommend it due to its hydration benefits. If you're interested in learning more about this, check out the 'Supplements' section in the 'Resources' chapter.

If you are a coffee drinker, I also recommend waiting for at least 1-hour after waking up to consume your coffee. So, if you wake up at 8:00 am, drink your mineral water and get your coffee to go, waiting to consume it until 9:00 am. You are allowed to have 1-2 small servings of cream in your coffee. And when I say cream, I mean half and half or something similar. You are not allowed to have any sugary-flavored creamers or any sugar-free creamers either. Basically, you are allowed to have a small amount of fat in your coffee and nothing more.

If you are hungry during the mid-morning, try having a carbonated beverage, like La-Croix or Perrier. These drinks can help reduce your hunger cravings. Make sure you consume drinks that have zero calories and zero sweeteners. The drinks mentioned above are perfect examples.

HOW YOU BREAK YOUR FAST: "THE FAST BREAK"

So, you've lasted until noon for the first day of controlled fasting. Congratulations if you've made it here! Now, it's time to break the fast. The way you beak your fast is very important. Your body is primed for nutrient uptake just as a high-performance race car. When the high-performance car runs out of fuel, you always make sure you use the high-octane (best fuel) to replenish what the car has used, right? Your body is no different. The quality of the fuel will mean the difference in performance immediately and especially over time.

Before you start eating, take this 'fast break' shake. It's simple, fast, and I believe it's very beneficial for setting you up for success and ideal for improved overall health.

There are two different ways you can employ the fast break.

1. Mix everything up in a small blender and knock it back.

2. Take the shot of apple cider separately. (this is my preferred way)

INGREDIENT 1: SPRING WATER (OR FILTERED WATER)

Water will serve two purposes: aiding digestion and contributing to your satiety. Water lubricates your joints, cushions your spinal cord, brain, and connective tissue, flushes body waste, helps maintain healthy blood pressure, etc. It also helps give you a feeling of fullness. Water fills your gut and you'll be less hungry. The less hungry you are, the easier it is to stay on point during all periods of time-restricted eating periods and controlled fasting periods. Remember: No diet, no matter how good it is, will cease to defy the physiological nature of the body. You have to create a calorie deficit if you want to burn fat. (In the full program, muscle building is another story and we will cover that in the chapters to come.)

Dose: 24 oz or 3/4 L.

INGREDIENT 2: 1/8 TSP OF PINK HIMALAYAN SEA SALT

We've discussed the benefits of pink Himalayan sea salt already, so no need to go in-depth here. However, it's great for breaking your fast due to the mineral content you're replacing in your body.

Dose: 1/4 tsp.

INGREDIENT 3: LEMON WATER

Lemons contain the following:

Hesperidin: A bioflavonoid that may help blood vessels function better. It may also reduce inflammation.

Citric acid: An antioxidant that protects the body from damaging free radicals.

Diosmin: Helpful for treating various disorders of blood vessels and protects against liver toxicity.

Eriocitrin: A lipid (fat) lowering properties in liver cells. It's also one of the plant pigments that gives lemons their color.

Pectin: A form of soluble fiber that's been shown to help with high cholesterol, high triglycerides, and to prevent colon cancer and prostate cancer.

Good sources of soluble fiber can help improve gut health, aid digestion, and keep blood sugar stable. This can help with weight loss, overall health, and I believe it serves as a perfect primer for breaking your fast.

Dose: 1 tbsp juice or 1/2 lemon, blended. (Some guys recommend only consuming the lemon juice and that's okay. You are certainly welcome to do this. However, consuming the pulp of the lemon is what provides you many of the added benefits.)

INGREDIENT 4: APPLE CIDER VINEGAR

Apple cider vinegar can help stimulate the digestive system without releasing insulin. It improves overall health, helps eliminate shitty bacteria, and balances healthy levels of pH in your stomach. It even stabilizes your blood sugar levels! You want to consume something that primes the pump, so you'll be in the perfect place to absorb all the good fuel you're about to consume—and apple cider vinegar is a hell of a solution!

Dose: 1 tsp.

(OPTIONAL) INGREDIENT 5: KAGED MUSCLE HYDRA CHARGE

Hydra Charge is one of my favorite supplements because it tastes so damn good. To me, it makes water more enjoyable to drink. When I like the taste of something, obviously, I'm going to be inclined to drink more of it. Hydra Charge contains 5 essential electrolytes from coconut water, taurine and SPECTRA, designed to support antioxidant potential. The reason I'm recommending it here is because of the aided hydration qualities I believe it provides and great taste. However, you certainly are not required to use it.

Dose: 1 scoop.

As I stated above, there are two ways you can do the Fast Break. I'll go more in depth here:

METHOD 1: MIX IT ALL UP IN A BLENDER (AND TAKE A SHOT OF APPLE CIDER VINEGAR SEPARATELY).

Here's how I do it: I add the water, salt, lemon and Hydra Charge to a small blender (I have a ninja blender and, if you're curious, here's a link for where you can find one like I use: LINK TO NINJA BLENDER). I'll blend it for 20-30 seconds with a few cubes of ice. After it's done, I'll get some apple cider vinegar out, take it like a shot of tequila, and chase it with my blended shake.

METHOD 2: MIX EVERYTHING UP AND DRINK IT ALL TOGETHER. (This is not my preferred way because apple cider vinegar has such a strong taste to me, I feel like it makes the whole shake much tougher to choke down. Kris does it this way, though. So, if you're tough as he is, go for this option!)

That's the Fast Break in its entirety. Most people consume this in a shake as do I. These steps might sound like a pain in the ass, especially because you have to blend the lemon.

However, it's doable and I really think it helps with everything you're doing!

After you drink your 'fast break' shake, it's time to eat!

The order of the types of food you eat are important. Below, please find the order in which you're supposed to consume different kinds of food. Trust me, it's less complicated than you think.

Order of food to be eaten:

1: Raw vegetables.

2: Cooked vegetables.

3: Protein.

4: Carbohydrates or fat.

As we already said, you've fasted for 12-hours and your body is primed and ready for nutrient uptake. In this fasted state, your body is like a sponge ready to ingest and utilize any fuel you give it. So choosing the appropriate fuel is of extreme importance for the following reasons:

1: Raw vegetables usually have the most nutrients compared to other foods. Get these in first and you'll notice improved energy, strength, and overall well-being. Your digestive system will act fast to break down the nutrients and turn it into usable energy.

2: Raw vegetables usually contain high amounts of fiber. Fiber not only aids in digestion but it also provides you a feeling of satiety (feeling of fullness). When you're trying to lose fat, remember you need to create a calorie deficit—you have to eat less than your body burns. When you eat less, you're almost always going to experience a sense of increased hunger. When you're hungry all the time, you obviously want to eat all the time. When you eat all the time, you're going to gain more weight/body fat. Eating more fiber in your diet makes you feel full and you'll be less likely to eat more food this way.

In his book 'The Warrior Diet', Ori Hofmekler describes breaking his fast with subtle tasting foods like raw vegetables and encourages the inclusion of as many different textures and colors as you can. I agree with this recommendation and encourage you to explore using foods that you enjoy and experiment with new flavors and textures when you break your fast.

Here's an example of how I break my fast. After the 'fast break' shake, I'll prepare a salad consisting of the following ingredients:

4-6 oz of grilled chicken
Baby spinach
Romaine
Arugula
Red onion
Green onion
Sliced red bell pepper
Sliced cucumber
Carrots
Celery
Tomatoes
Sugar snap peas

I also throw in a small amount* of salad topping ingredients like:

Bacon bits
Wonton strips
Tortilla strips
Dried cranberries
etc.

*For these, I use a minimal amount, which adds a lot of taste and makes for one epic salad. For dressing, I use vinegar or balsamic vinegar. Also, a note on seasonings: I don't skimp on salt, either. I like salt and pepper as well as seasoned salt.

RULE: For meals in the afternoon and evening, remember the following: *Always drink 1 glass of water and eat veggies with each meal.*

What types of meals can you eat? Just about anything you would normally eat. Just make sure you add veggies. Try to eat healthy, of course. This means try to avoid eating out and stay away from fast food restaurants.

For your eating window, try and space your meals a few hours apart. That being said, you can have as many meals during this time as you like. If you break your fast at noon, your next meals will be 3:00 pm and 6:00 pm respectively. Personally, I prefer to have 2 or 3 meals evenly spaced apart during my feeding window during this Primer Phase. I like doing it this way due to its simplicity and convenience.

When you are done eating for the day, try to make sure this last meal is consumed within 2-hours before bedtime. Doing this allows your digestive system ample time to work on processing your food and passing it to your small intestine. So, by the time you jump in bed, your body has had the chance to process the last meal of the day. The idea to stop eating 2-hours before bedtime also relates to our circadian rhythm. In the evening, our body starts preparing for rest by producing melatonin, a sleep hormone. In a recent study, 110 college students aged 18-22 were observed for a 30-day sleep-wake period.

"Researchers assessed meals, calories consumed, and their timing against sleep, activity and body fat. They noticed that for individuals with higher body fat, the midpoint of all the calories they consumed for the day was later than for leaner people, and 1 hour closer to the onset of melatonin release."

https://www.ncbi.nlm.nih.gov/pubmedhealth/behindtheheadlines/news/2017-09-12-avoid-eating-just-before-your-bedtime-study-recommends/

There are various studies showing people who eat immediately before bed have a higher probability of gaining more weight.

https://www.ncbi.nlm.nih.gov/pubmed/25439026

https://www.ncbi.nlm.nih.gov/pubmed/23814334

The practice of avoiding food at least 2-hours before bedtime gives our digestive system a break and serves our circadian rhythm more positively. When it's time to sleep, you want to take advantage of the most optimal strategy designed to get the best bang for the buck. Interfering with your circadian rhythm isn't your best bet.

[The primer week should give you basic understanding of fasting and how to deal with hunger and satiety. Knowing your body and how it responds to different instances will give you a better frame of reference as it relates to fasting and health in general.]

PUTTING IT ALL TOGETHER

Rules of the Primer Phase:

The goal is to fast 12-hours each day. (For most people, you usually won't start eating until 12:00 pm.)

During your controlled fasting period, try to make it though it without eating anything. However, you are allowed to have some calories during this time. For example, you can have trace amounts of creamer with your coffee and/or a pre-workout supplement if you work out in the morning.

Consume the 'fast break' shake before you start eating your first meal.

For your first meal after the fast break, try eating a salad and include as many different textures and colors as possible.

For other meals:

Drink 1 glass of water with each meal.
Eat veggies with each meal.
Try and space meals a few hours apart if you can.
Try and finish eating your final meal of the day 2-hours before bedtime.

FAQ Section for Primer Phase:

Q: What if I work nights?

A: It doesn't matter what time you work. Just skip your first meal and begin eating in the middle of 'your day'. For example, if you're a hospital worker, your day would start like this:

7:00 pm: Wake up

9:00 pm: Begin work

12:00 am: Assuming this is your lunchtime, you'd begin eating your first meal here. Eat your meals like normal (including the rules above).

11:00 am: Assuming you'd go to bed at this time, stop eating at 9:00 am or earlier.

Q: When do I work out during this primer week?

A: It doesn't matter. Whatever time is most convenient will work.

Q: Can I drink anything else during my fasting window in the mornings?

A: Yes. You can drink coffee with small amounts of cream if you wish.

Q: If I'm seeing results with the Primer Phase, is it okay to keep doing it?

A: Of course. This week is a form of time-restricted eating and will help you get in shape. In my opinion, it's perfectly fine to eat this way all the time, if you wish.

Q: Can I have any other food during my fast?

A: No. For this week, we're only fasting for a few hours after we wake up. You can do this, right? It's only a few hours! Lol.

Q: What about supplements? Can I have any during my fast?

A: Yes and no. During this week, you can use supplements that contain little to no calories. Pre-workouts like Kaged Muscle Pre-Kaged works great. If you lift in the am, go ahead and take a pre-workout. Other supplements that are okay: Anything that doesn't contain a lot of carbs (Less than 10g of carbs). Examples that are okay:

BCAAs (example: Kaged Muscle's BCAA Powder, Pre-Kaged, or In-Kaged)

Intra-workout products (example: Kaged Muscle In-Kaged).

Hydrating products (example: Kaged Muscle Hydra Charge).

Supplements not to take during this fasted window: Protein powders, high-carb powders, etc. The idea is to keep calories low during the fasting window. Just look at the labels of products to confirm. As a rule of thumb: If it has more than 10g of carbs, 10g of protein, or 10g of fat per serving, don't use it during your fasting window. You can take these types of products after you break your controlled fast.

THE ACCLIMATION PHASE

During this phase of controlled fasting, small adjustments will be made to your time-restricted eating schedule and help you gain an even better understanding of how fasting works. FYI: This will continue to get a little more difficult during each phase. Just remember: You're not depriving yourself of anything. For the most part, you aren't changing WHAT you eat. You are simply changing the TIMES you eat.

Do you think you're ready? If so, let's get into it.

This week, you aren't going to start eating until the afternoon. Have I scared you yet? Don't worry—it's not that bad. We are going to follow the similar rules as The Primer Phase with a few modifications.

Day One - Day Three: Begin eating your first meal in the mid-afternoon. In a sense, you're going to skip breakfast and lunch. Drink 20 oz of water immediately after you wake up in the morning. It's okay to have coffee with trace amounts of cream. If you are starving and just can't take it, it's okay to have a whey protein shake in the mid-morning (example: Kaged Muscle Re-Kaged).

(Remember, we are implementing a 'controlled fasting' protocol. This means we are eating little to no food during the under-eating phase. During a water fast, you wouldn't eat anything. The only thing you'd consume is water. I bring this up because it's a very popular question.)

Try to drink as much water as you can during the day. Once you make it to your mid-afternoon feeding window, you're going to begin your meal with a salad, just as you did during The Primer Phase. Try to include as many different colors and textures as possible. It's okay to include any meat you like (i.e. whole eggs, chicken, steak, fish, etc.). For protein amounts, follow the following suggestion: For males, aim for 6-8 oz of protein. For females, aim for 4-5 oz of protein. You are free to eat more protein if you like, just make sure you eat at least 6 oz for men and 4 oz for women.

For the meal or two following, drink 20 oz of water before you eat. Include veggies as well. Stop eating your last meal of the day at least 2-hours before bedtime.

IN SUMMARY, THE ACCLIMATION PHASE BREAKS DOWN AS FOLLOWS:

Don't start eating until mid-afternoon (preferably 2:00 pm or 3:00 pm).

Drink a glass of water with each meal.

First meal: eat a salad and include as many different colors and textures as possible.

All other meals: eat the foods you'd normally eat BUT include veggies.

Protein in each meal: Eat at least 6 oz for men and 4 oz for women.

Drink 1 glass of water with each meal (and it's suggested that you try and drink around 1 gallon of water by end the day).

Eat veggies with each meal.

Try and space meals a few hours apart if you can.

Try and finish eating your final meal of the day 2-hours before bedtime.

FAQ Section for Acclimation Phase:

Q: I'm starving and don't think I can go this whole week waiting to eat my first meal until the afternoon. Can I go back to having my first meal in the middle of the day instead of afternoon?

A: Yes. You are still trying to get used to fasting and how your body is reacting to these new changes. If you find it too difficult to wait until the afternoon to start eating, you can go back to eating your first meal at noon. However, I'd like you to follow the rules for The Acclimation Phase for at least 3-days before you go back to eating at noon. Remember, you're feeling hunger pains because your body is not used to going this long without eating. But guess what? Your body is turning up its fat burning capabilities and autophagy (cell cleansing). If you can follow this protocol, I am very confident you are going to love the results. You want to feel better and look better? Stay true to the plan and keep working hard. Nothing worth having is easy. You can do this!

Q: When do I work out during this acclimation week?

A: It doesn't matter. Whatever time is most convenient will work.

Q: Can I drink anything else during my fasting window in the mornings?

A: Yes. You can drink coffee with small amounts of cream if you wish.

Q: Can I have any other food during my fast?

A: Yes. You can have veggies and one whey protein shake (aim for not consuming more than 30g of protein though). The idea is to keep your food consumption amounts small. We want to fire up your body's thermogenesis (fat burning) and improve your health. Giving your digestive system a break is the name of the game.

That's it! Really, the only difference between the Primer Phase and the Acclimation Phase is adjusting the periods of time-restricted eating windows. The theories taught in the Fasting Plan are simple. But they aren't necessarily easy. With the full program, you won't ever see complex instructions that aren't easy to internalize. The goal in developing this program has and always will be: To get you positive results in your health and appearance that stay with you throughout your life! We are about to change who we are for who we will become!

THE FAT BURNING FASTING PLAN

Once you've completed the Primer Phase and the Acclimation Phase, you're now ready to begin the Fat Burning Fasting Plan. You're used to fasting and have a good idea of what to expect. We will start with a cycle of controlled fasting combining the following forms:

22/2 OR 20/4 CONTROLLED INTERMITTENT FASTING

16/8 CONTROLLED INTERMITTENT FASTING

Day One - Day Four: We will be implementing the 22/2 Controlled Intermittent Fasting Technique. Since most people begin their week on Monday, we will start with this day. However, it doesn't matter which day of the week you begin the Fat Burning Protocol. Remember that controlled fasting consists of eating little to no calories during the day. I've found that people work better when they have specific guidelines, so the rules are as follows:

Rule 1: Eat no more than 200 calories during the controlled fasting window.

Rule 2: You must drink ¾ - 1 gallon of water during the controlled fasting window.

*Follow these rules 100 percent. No questions. No exceptions.

Here's how the day will break down:

In our example, the program starts on Monday. You'll have your last meal on Sunday night. On Monday morning, you'll wake up and begin your controlled fasting time period. The plan is to fast all day by eating little to no food. But, if you are starving, you are allowed to have some veggies. I also prefer to have trace amounts of creamer in my coffee because I enjoy it.

Your day will start like this:

Wake up and follow the morning routine:

5:30 am: Wake up and drink the 'fast break' shake

*'Fast Break' Shake consisting of:

20-24 oz of spring water
1/4 lemon
1/8 tsp of pink Himalayan sea salt
Optional
1 scoop of Kaged Muscle Hydra Charge
1 scoop of Kaged Muscle L-Glutamine
1 tsp of organic turmeric

5:45 am: Activity

Studies have shown that getting your blood moving in the morning upon waking up can improve your thermogenesis during the day. Here is a very brief workout that will get your heart rate up and will set you up for success. Try the following routine which should only take you 5-10 minutes. If you can't perform 100 push-ups in a row, complete as many as you can and rest for 15-30 seconds. Keep pushing out reps and resting until you complete all 100 reps.

1-   100 Push-ups
2-   20 Burpees
3-   3 Sets of 30 crunches with bands

8:00 am: Start working and have more water

9:00 am: Coffee with cream

10:30 am: Sparkling water

*2:00 pm: Small veggie meal

If you are starving your ass off and don't think you'll make it until the evening 'feeding window", go ahead and eat a vegetable tray with a low-fat ranch dressing or hummus. If you can make it without eating this meal, that is optimal. A decent time to do this is anywhere from 12:00 pm to 2:00 pm.

An example is:

1 sliced red bell pepper
100g of sugar snap peas
10 carrots
50g of cauliflower
1 sliced tomato

5:00 PM: Consume Pre-Workout with 20-24 oz of water

5:30 PM: Workout

7-7:30 PM: Time to eat

IF YOU WORK OUT IN THE AM:

If you work out in the morning, go ahead and hit the gym. If you take a pre-workout, go ahead and drink it with another 20 oz of water 30-minutes before hitting the gym. I recommend Pre-Kaged by Kaged Muscle Supplements. Since this program implements controlled fasting instead of water fasting, you will have little to no food during your fasting (time-restricted eating) window. This is why you can have pre-workout supplements and/or small amounts of certain foods and drinks.

After you're the finished workout, drink more water. For taste, you can add lemon to it.

If you are absolutely starving after the gym, you are allowed to have a small whey protein shake with water (no more than 30g of protein). If you can make it without the whey protein, go for it. Having protein powder isn't necessary in my opinion. Since our goal in this chapter is to burn as much fat as possible, we are going to do everything we can to maximize our body's dependence on using stored fat as energy instead of glycogen. The lower amount of food we ingest will also help promote autophagy (cell-cleansing) and aid in helping improve our insulin sensitivity.

The rest of the day, the point is to avoid food and focus on work. This is your time-restricted eating window. During the morning hours, you will be the hungriest—understanding this, you can have coffee with trace amounts of creamer (half and half is okay but stay away from the sugar-free creamers and other sugary creamers).

You can also have sparkling water beverages, like Perrier, Pellegrino, and La-Croix. These are great because they help curb your hunger and are pretty tasty.

The above are only examples. You can also combine these into a small salad. The idea is to eat a good amount of veggies you enjoy until you have a full feeling. But try not to overdo it. Eating veggies or having whey protein won't necessarily affect your progress, but if you get to the point where you don't need any food, you will have more control over your body and mind. This will help you turn this program into a way of life. If you can stick to this, guess what? You're going to get lean and stay lean all year long as I have.

THE FEEDING WINDOW:

After you've fasted during the day, it's time to finally eat. This is where the fun begins. Usually, I choose to eat around 6:00 or 7:00 pm if I've worked out in the morning. I don't set a specific time. However, I focus on trying to fast as long as possible during the day to give my body a chance to burn fat and detoxify. Usually, the time-restricted period of eating lasts around 20-22 hours. (Hence the names '20/4' and '22/2').

For the Fasting Plan, every time you break your fast, you are instructed to perform the Fast Break (discussed in chapter 6).

After you employ the Fast Break, the order of foods to be eaten is important. Refer to the directions below.

ORDER OF FOODS TO BE EATEN:

You've fasted for most of the day and your body is primed and ready for nutrient uptake. In this fasted state, your body is like a sponge ready to ingest and utilize any fuel you give it.

So choosing the appropriate fuel is of extreme importance. Here's the order of food to be eaten:

1: Raw vegetables

2: Cooked vegetables

3: Protein

4: Carbohydrates or fat

There are a few reasons why we recommend food to be eaten in this order:

1: Raw vegetables usually have the most nutrients compared to other foods. Get these in first and you'll notice improved energy, strength, and overall well-being. Your digestive system will act fast to break down the nutrients and turn it into usable energy.

2: Raw vegetables usually contain high amounts of fiber. Fiber not only aids in digestion but it also provides you a feeling of satiety (feeling of fullness). When you're trying to lose fat, remember you need to create a calorie deficit—you have to eat less than your body burns. When you eat less, you're almost always going to experience a sense of increased hunger. When you're hungry all the time, you obviously want to eat all the time. When you eat all the time, you're going to gain more weight/body-fat. Eating more fiber in your diet makes you feel full and you'll be less likely to eat more food this way.

In his book 'The Warrior Diet', Ori Hofmekler describes breaking his fast with subtle tasting foods like raw vegetables and encourages the inclusion of as many different textures and colors as you can. I agree with this recommendation and encourage you to explore using foods that you enjoy and experiment with new flavors and textures when you break your fast. I've also found that eating food in the order described above will give you better results because you'll eat the nutrient-dense foods first, giving your body a higher grade of fuel. The fiber from the nutrient-dense foods will also give you a better feeling of satiety. The more full you are, the less likely you are to overeat. See what I'm getting at here? Magic pills aren't the answer and they don't exist anyway. Systematically planned ways of eating

The following is an example of how I break my fast. First, I'll have the 'fast break' shake. Then, I'll make myself the following salad:

1c spinach
1c romaine lettuce
1 sliced bell pepper
Half cucumber
1/4c corn
1/2c blueberries
1/4c cherry tomatoes
Vinegar for dressing

While I'm eating my salad, I'll grill some asparagus on the barbecue, adding some non-fat cooking spray and garlic salt.

For protein, I'll grill some flank steak or petite sirloin. I prefer cuts that are lean. Sometimes, I'll have rice with the steak and other times I'll have a baked potato (white or sweet potato).

Above is only an example. The main goal is to eat veggies first and follow it up with protein and carbs. Experiment with the food that you enjoy the most. Refer to the list of nutrient-dense foods at the beginning of this chapter if you need more ideas. I've also included a 'Recipe' section at the end of the book in the 'References' section for your convenience.

Eat your dinner and enjoy yourself. This is the time to eat as much as you like with no guilt. Eating food in that order is optimal because it fuels your body with fiber, vitamins and other great stuff before you eat everything else. In a fasted state, your body is in a perfect position to partition nutrients into your muscle as opposed to fat.

Pay attention to your hunger and thirst as you eat. Once you become more thirsty than you are hungry, stop eating for 20-30 minutes. I have to thank Ori Hofmekler for this great tip. In his book 'The Warrior Diet', he recommends the same. However, he likes to wait 10-15 minutes in this state and I prefer to wait longer to give my body a better chance to digest what I've eaten.

Above is how the 20-4 fast is done. You will do the 20-4 fast Monday through Thursday (or 4-days per week if you start on a different day).

On Friday and Saturday, you will employ a 16-8 fast. Try to schedule your eating window between 12:00 pm and 8:00 pm if you can. I've found this is the most convenient and the most effective. These days will be similar to what you did during the Primer Phase. Just remember to fast for 16-hours.

RULES FOR THE FAT BURNING PROTOCOL:

20/4: Fast for 20-hours. Eat during a 4-hour window.

16/8: Fast for 16-hours. Eat during an 8-hour window.

Drink this morning shake everyday upon waking: Consume 24 oz of room temperature water with pink Himalayan sea salt. (Optional: Add Kaged Muscle Hydra Charge for taste.)

Wait 1-hour after waking up to consume coffee (can have trace amounts of cream if you like).

If you're hungry in mid-morning, you can have sparkling water (a zero calorie, zero sweetener, carbonated beverage).

Eat no more than 200 calories during your fasting period.

Consume the 'fast break' shake before you start eating your first meal.

For your first meal after the fast break, try eating a salad and include as many different textures and colors as possible.

For other meals:

Drink 1 glass of water with each meal.

Eat veggies with each meal.

Try and space meals a few hours apart if you can.

Try and finish eating your final meal of the day 2-hours before bedtime.

On the last day of the week, you'll eat as you normally would. You won't be fasting. This day will serve as a re-feed day. I like to call it a 'reset day'. Over the years of my fitness competition days, I used a lot of methods of dieting. One of my favorites was carb cycling. This simply means you'd adjust carbohydrate amounts during the week while keeping your body in a deficit to burn fat. An example would be to eat low carbs Monday through Thursday, medium amounts of carbs on Friday and Saturday, and follow it up with a high day on Sunday. This helped me burn fat and primed me for the fitness show by giving me an idea of how my body would react to higher amounts of carbs. This idea is called glycogen supercompensation. Bodybuilders have used this form of dieting for years to burn fat and it's been very successful for them. Without going to in-depth, your body gets fuel from carbohydrates and stores them in your muscle as glycogen. This is what gives your muscles the full look. The rest is stored in your liver. When you strip yourself from carbs for long enough periods of time, your body will look flat and depleted. You'll burn high amounts of fat in this state, but you'll look and feel like shit. Since your body has been depleted, it soaks up carbs like a sponge when you reintroduce them into your diet. It's said that your body might hold as much as 2 to 2.5 times the normal amounts of glycogen. This is why they call it 'glycogen supercompensation'.

This was great when I did shows because it helped me get leaner while giving me an idea of what my body would look like after being super compensated with glycogen. Each week, as I would get leaner, I would be able to tighten up and tweak the amount of carbs I'd need to look my best for the show.

This idea of carb cycling led me to throw around the idea of cycling the types of fasting for better results. This is how the fasting plan was born. Cycling the different types of fasting days, followed with a re-feed day (reset day), would provide you with a significant advantage of fat burning. The reset day has proven itself to be a great addition as well. While I haven't performed studies on this type of cycling, I have had lots of personal success with this type of fasting as well as many of my clients. I'm saying this to you because I love this stuff and I'd like you to know how I've stumbled upon this technique and I'm eager to hear your feedback. So far, the results have been incredible!

TO SUMMARIZE, THE FAT BURNING PROTOCOL WILL BREAK DOWN AS FOLLOWS:

Monday through Thursday: 20-4 Fast

Friday and Saturday: 16-8 Fast

Sunday: Reset Day

Repeat everything again the next week. I've been living this lifestyle for a longtime. It's very simple and reproducible, allowing for strong flexibility. This makes it easier to adhere to—and remember: The keys to every successful program starts with adherence.

That concludes The Fat Burning Protocol. I look forward to seeing amazing things from you!

Thank you for checking this out! Please keep me updated on your progress by tagging me in your social media. The most rewarding thing I get back is seeing the difference you make in your life! I mean that with my heart and soul. Seeing you succeed makes this ALL WORTH IT!

"The only way to make sense out of change is to plunge into it, move with it, and join the dance."

Alan Watts

About The Author

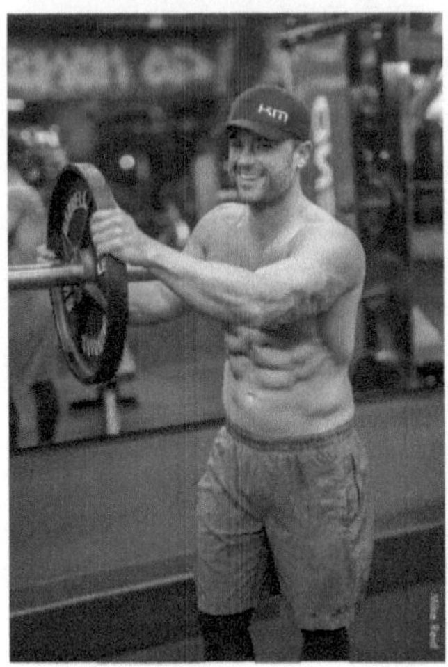

My name is Nick Holt.

I've spent over 20 years of my life lifting weights and competing in fitness competitions. I've tried just about every different type of diet there is. My goal has never been to become a 300lb bodybuilder nor has it been to become a professional fitness model. Nope. I wanted to be in the NBA.

I begin my career in fitness at age 11 when I picked up my first basketball and, from that moment, I had been hooked on becoming the best ball player I could be. I'd even sneak into the local gym to work on my game until my parents finally broke down and bought a membership for me. To get better at basketball, I started lifting weights. I started noticing new improvements in my basketball skills and a few girls took notice of my abs that started forming. This led to more confidence and I started reading bodybuilding magazines and learning more about fitness. At 20 years old, I began competing in fitness competitions like bodybuilding and, eventually, men's physique.

The more competitions I did, the more I started realizing something. What was going on? I wanted to add more muscle and I knew that in order to do this, I needed to eat more food. But I started to use this as an excuse to justify eating poorly. When I was training for shows, I'd spend 2-3 nights each week cooking my meals of chicken, broccoli, and brown rice and packing them in Tupperware. Each day, I'd lug a cooler around with me that included 6 meals of frozen food and eat every 2-3 hours. During this time, I was lean and shredded.

After the show season ended, I'd switch to building mode and try and add muscle to my frame, so I'd place better in competitions. During this time, I'd still prepare my meals in advance and hit the gym just as hard. However, I'd also use the off-season as an excuse to eat more junk food, drink a little, and spend more social time with friends. During shows, I'd be lean and shredded. During the off-season, I looked chubby.

When I'd start noticing myself putting on more weight than planned, I'd pick a show and start preparing for it by leaning down. I started noticing myself using shows as a justifiable excuse to actually 'get in shape' and not be fat. I don't like feeling chubby. No one does. So, I wondered if there was a way to obtain what I feel is a perfect body for me and keep that perfect body year-round?

The idea of improving has always appealed to me. From the moment I picked up my first weight at 13 years old, I have been interested in finding a way to obtain the perfect physique. This led to a never-ending amount of experiences with vast amounts of dieting programs and tactics that have ultimately led me to write this program about fasting and share my experiences with you, so you can do the same thing I've done which is to get lean and stay lean all year long.

Learn more about me and the fasting plan at www.thefastingplan.com.

ONE LAST THING...

If you enjoyed this book or found it useful I'd be very grateful if you'd post a short review on Amazon. Your support really does make a difference and I read all the reviews personally so I can get your feedback and make this book even better.

If you'd like to leave a review then all you need to do is click the review link on this book's page on Amazon

Thanks again for your support!